*The International Library of Psychology*

# THE CAVEMAN WITHIN US

*Founded by C. K. Ogden*

# The International Library of Psychology

## GENERAL PSYCHOLOGY
### In 38 Volumes

# THE CAVEMAN WITHIN US

## His Peculiarities and Powers; How We Can Enlist His Aid for Health and Efficiency

WILLIAM J FIELDING

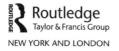
Routledge
Taylor & Francis Group

NEW YORK AND LONDON

First published in 1922 by
Kegan Paul, Trench, Trubner & Co., Ltd.

Reprinted in 1999 by
Routledge
2 Park Square, Milton Park, Abingdon, Oxon, OX14 4RN
711 Third Avenue, New York, NY 10017

*Routledge is an imprint of the Taylor & Francis Group*

First issued in paperback 2013

Transferred to Digital Printing 2006

The publishers have made every effort to contact authors/copyright holders
of the works reprinted in the *International Library of Psychology*.
This has not been possible in every case, however, and we would
welcome correspondence from those individuals/companies
we have been unable to trace.

These reprints are taken from original copies of each book. In many cases
the condition of these originals is not perfect. The publisher has gone to
great lengths to ensure the quality of these reprints, but wishes to point
out that certain characteristics of the original copies will, of necessity, be
apparent in reprints thereof.

*British Library Cataloguing in Publication Data*
A CIP catalogue record for this book
is available from the British Library

ISBN13: 978-0-415-21015-7 (hbk)

ISBN13: 978-0-415-85280-7 (pbk)

# CONTENTS

# CONTENTS

# CONTENTS

# INTRODUCTION

It is generally agreed that the great preponderance of human ills and ailments is due to disturbances of a neurotic character. The effects of these disturbances are so manifold and far-reaching that the real seat of the trouble is often obscured by the physical symptoms. Because these symptoms may express themselves through any organ, muscle or portion of the body, and simulate almost any known malady, the problem is an exceedingly intricate, and frequently a baffling one.

So-called "nervous exhaustion," neurasthenia and other neuroses of various types and degrees of morbidity are conceded to be the diseases most typical of our civilization. Notwithstanding their supremacy in the domain of pathology, it is the purpose of this book to show that these "nervous" afflictions are not in any way the inevitable result of cultural progress, but rather that they are excrescences to be avoided. Even more specifically, it is the object of this work to demonstrate *how* they may be avoided.

These subtle and sinister disorders are in reality maladjustments of the mechanism of personality. They indicate a lack of coördination between the primitive and cultural components of our nature. They represent a struggle between the Caveman and the Socialized Being. Paradoxically, these two constituents are one and indivisible, merged into a single organism, and yet each is as real in the distinctive characteristics that it manifests as though the span of a hundred thousand years separated their existence.

When two such heterogeneous factors—each with innate tendencies peculiar to itself—are incorporated into a single organic entity, it is evident than an intelligent understanding of the mechanism as a whole is not only desirable, but absolutely necessary, for internal harmony and efficient operation.

It is because of the necessity for realizing the importance of the human being's great primitive heritage as a dominant influence in the present, that I have stressed this phase of the subject, particularly in Chapter II. In order to obtain a true picture of the personality, it is essential that it should be shown in the perspective of its immense biological background.

Naturally, the researches of the psychoanalytic school have been drawn upon and the fundamental psychic laws brought into their proper relation with the findings of the experimental physiologists, and all of these are correlated with the accepted hypotheses of the leading biologists and anthropologists. The result is a many-sided view of the human organism, with all its dynamic ramifications.

But a complete exposition of the personality is hardly possible by setting forth merely the vital facts of biology, psychology and physiology. It is equally important to show the reactions of the inherent emotional nature to social phenomena, and to fulfil this requirement I have drawn upon a wealth of historical and biographical material.

Throughout the entire period of history and, from what we may infer, long before that time, no phase of man's social life has found so rich a field for expression as the religious. Because the history of mankind has been woven into the warp and woof of innumerable supernatural beliefs, all of which, however, have so much in common, it is fitting that a chapter should be devoted to the appeal of religion to the emotional or primitive side of man.

Both ancient and modern man has been dominated by popular prejudices concerning his social traditions, his accepted ideas and ideals, and the prevailing institutions of his particular period. His emotional reaction to these social phenomena his given us, and continues to give us, epochs of witch-hunting, heresy-hunting, persecution for unorthodox ideas, tyrannous exhibitions of the crowd-spirit no less than of the autocrat, mass and class mobs, race riots and pogroms, puritanical obsessions and wholesale inhibitions. An understanding of these universal convulsive expressions is as necessary to an insight into the mechanism of personality as is a knowledge of the elementary facts of biology.

The two extremes in the gamut of human possibilities have been analyzed for the purpose of demonstrating that, *under the cultural veneer,* all human beings are essentially alike. The duality of personality is the unvarying law.

In the chapter on Genius, it will be seen that the world's greatest luminaries have revealed, behind their compelling brilliancy, a basically primitive human organism, which so often has reflected itself in their character and conduct. Not infrequently has the Caveman broken out in all his primordial abandon. Everywhere in the realm of Genius, he is in evidence. And from these peaks of human attainment down to the lowlands of halted development and chronic immaturity, there is the inevitable contrast in each individual of the primitive and the socialized nature. Only in the relative proportion of social adaptation is there endless variation.

As the possibility for individual happiness and health is bound up irretrievably with the question of environment, it will be perceived why social factors of necessity have been stressed. Too much importance cannot be laid on an understanding of one's relation to the powerful social forces that constitute the dynamics of environment.

When an individual has grasped the fact of the essential *duality of his nature*—and it is the intention that this book, by analyzing and clarifying so much of the mechanism of personality, will enable him clearly to *visualize* this phenomenon—he will have acquired the insight requisite to Self-understanding. He will understand the psychic and physical processes of the machine he is trying to run.

With this key to Self-understanding in his possession, he will be able to open the doors of Self-mastery and Self-expression. This means an undreamed of freedom from the myriad forms of so-called nervous afflictions, with their far-reaching symptoms of physical disability, and the achievement of a new and greater measure of health and efficiency.

WILLIAM J. FIELDING.

# THE CAVEMAN
# WITHIN US

# THE CAVEMAN WITHIN US

---

# CHAPTER I

## THE CAVEMAN AND THE MODERN—OUR DUAL NATURE

> This same human nature's a singular thing;
> It sticks to people so strangely long.
>
>   •    •    •    •    •    •
>
> I thought to myself the old Adam, for certain,
> Had for good and all been kicked out of doors;
> But lo! in two shakes he's atop again.
> Ay ay, my son, we must treat you, I see,
> To cure this pestilent human nature.
>       —IBSEN, *The Old Man* in ''Peer Gynt.''

THAT every individual possesses a well-defined dual nature is now a thoroughly established scientific fact. There is elaborate physiological and psychological proof—in other words, incontrovertible biological evidence—to sustain this contention.

You may not like it—or you may not particularly care. If you object to the allegation that you are not entirely (but only partly) the ethical, law-abiding James Henry Jones that you are reputed to be, then yours should be the pleasure of disproving the charge without trouble after you have perused the argument.

If you think you are not sufficiently interested or concerned whether you are or not, then there may be even stronger reasons why you should know. No self-respecting human being should accept this charge with equanimity, and to know *why*, may enable you to understand, and to become acquainted with the Caveman within you—the factor that contributes so much to your real, all-around personality.

You are honest, loyal and altruistic—that is, on the surface; perhaps never have been in jail—but do you know that this Cave-creature within you is *at bottom* absolutely unethical, anti-social, egotistical, primitive, and otherwise destitute of all the cherished virtues?

In this respect, there is no cause for alarm. It merely proves you are human; neither more nor less. And by getting an insight into the situation, you will better be able to adjust yourself to the problems of life. It will become a valuable guide in pursuing your destiny, as necessary in present-day life as is the chart of the navigator on the high seas.

After all, despite his faults, this old troglodyte within us can be trained to cooperate and help us carry our burdens. It is true he is not intellectual or moral, but he is strong and robust. He is *vital.* If we allow him to dominate us, he will submerge us into the mire of a vicious or criminal existence.

If we attempt to suppress him, he will rebel with all his primitive might and throw us into the fitful arms of physical or mental sickness, thus adding another victim to the hosts of neurotics and diseased.

However, when reasonably disciplined, he has his channels of approach, such as catering to his love of amusement and fun, adventure, harmless vanities, and many other diversions that conform to the social proprieties.

The problem of making this adjustment is the most serious one of every individual's life. It decides his fate and possibilities for realizing happiness, in marriage and out; his capacity for achievement in his calling; his faculty to make friends and successfully "mix" in the heterogeneous composition of the community. The capacity for making this adjustment varies in each person, depending in a measure upon his inherent qualities and even to a larger extent upon his early environment, whether helpful and constructive or negative and depressive.

The dual nature of the human personality has been *sensed* by philosophers and others from remote antiquity. In its various manifestations, it is a constant theme in the folklore, legends and literature of all periods and all languages. It has been a cause of wonder, astonishment and chagrin. It has resulted in infinite distress, heart-pangs, and often disaster to the more immediate victims of its caprices. But it has been taken for granted, as a matter of course, without being understood. Anything not understood is a mystery, and the natural phenomena of life mantled in mystery have been the bugbear of the race in its long, struggling ascent.

### The Basis of Witchcraft

In centuries past, men and women who had shown too pronounced evidence of this dual trait of 'personality were said to be "possessed by devils," or "evil spirits." They had been "bewitched." Countless thousands have been burned at the stake, thrown into medieval prisons or otherwise penalized for their indiscretion in harbouring the damned. We still do homage to the memory of Old Mother Witch on Hallowe'en, and recount her exploits to our children as they listen to the fables of old.

It is true that the persecuted persons were exceptions, forming only a small minority of the population; but the ominous fact remains that almost anyone was a *possible* victim. No one knew but what his turn might come next to answer to the charge of witchcraft or some allied crime of sorcery. The prevalence of witch-hunting was, of course, much greater in some places than others. Some idea of the popularity of this form of diversion may be gained from the fact that within the course of a few years six thousand five hundred people were executed for witchcraft in the principality of Trèves alone.

And so, better to protect themselves against suspicion, men and women spied upon their neighbors, eagerly watching for any sign that could be construed as evidence of a visitation from sinister sources. Even within the family circle, the blight of this fanaticism was not unknown.

If, upon occasion, the squint of one's eye did not just conform to the ocular conventions (possibly "looking daggers"), there was danger of having to answer to the charge of possessing the "evil eye."

All of these occurrences denoted a recognition of some factor in the personality·that was considered *apart* from what was expected of the social or ethical human being. The fact that, at times, everyone felt certain impulses or urges to do the proscribed thing, tended to make most individuals compensate for this feeling of inner guilt by being the more anxious to find evidence of a similar failing in someone else. In this way the individual, by accusing another, felt himself strengthened, or raised to a higher plane. It took his attention and that of the community off his own shortcomings by focusing it on another.

In other words, instead of raising himself to a higher level by some creative or socially useful work or deed, he attempted to achieve superiority (and he actually experienced a genuine feeling of superiority) by lowering the prestige of others about him. This tendency did not die with the demise of popular belief in witchcraft. It is still universal, as I shall later demonstrate in numerous instances.

The old penalties for this misunderstood conduct were quite in accord with the methods used for meeting all other problems of an unknown or mysterious origin. Every phenomenon of this nature was considered either the will of God or the work of the Devil. If the former, there was the attitude to accept it as inevitable, the only hope being to make some reparation or supplication to appease the wrath of the Almighty. If the work of the Devil, the task was somewhat simpler. As the Devil, ever since the unfortunate Garden of Eden episode, has been accredited with the habit of operating through some animal or human agency, it was obviously a matter of laying hands on the culprit through whom his Satanic Majesty functioned, and prescribing a suitable penalty.

Certain symptoms which are well known to present-day physicians as an indication of hysteria were in the old days regarded as indisputable proof that the victim was a witch. One of these characteristic symptoms was the famous "devil's claw," a patch of insensitive skin somewhere upon the body of the alleged witch. This sign is frequently met in modern medical practice under the more reassuring designation of "hysterical anaesthesia." The establishing of the existence of the "devil's claw," in connection with other grotesque tests, constituted the procedure of the witch trial.

The early scriptural writings took cognizance of witchcraft, as we observe in the command given in *Exodus* (xxii—18) "Thou shalt not suffer a sorceress to live." Similar threats against witches, wizards, etc., frequently occur in Leviticus and Deuteronomy.

The most estimable people asserted the existence of witchcraft and warned against its practice. Says Sir William Blackstone: "To deny the possibility, nay, the actual existence of witchcraft and sorcery, is at once flatly to contradict the revealed Word of God in various passages of the Old and New Testaments, and the thing itself is a truth to which every nation in the world hath, in its turn, borne testimony, either by example seemingly well attested, or by prohibitory laws, which at least suppose the possibility of a commerce with evil spirits."

The Church at a very early period formally admitted its existence, and fulminated against all who practiced it. The fourth canon of the Council of Auxerre, in 525, strongly prohibited all resort to sorcerers, diviners, augurers, and the like.

As at the present time, those who refuse to follow the ' crowd are called various names to which is attached a popular odium, so in the days of witch-hunting, those who tried to discredit this feverish pastime were denounced as "Sadducees" and atheists.

### Primitive Reasoning

An apt illustration of the manner in which serious problems of an unknown origin were met may be observed in the case of plagues and epidemics. These periodic visitations of pestilence, which swept off whole sections of the population, were usually accepted as an act of divine retribution. No connection was seen between filth, or lack of sanitation, and disease. Before the dawn, and in the twilight, of modern science, every unknown scourge or misfortune was attributed to God, or His handy antithesis, the Devil.

To carry this process of primitive, illogical "reasoning" from social to individual or psychological problems, was but a step. In fact, the attitude that made one possible, made the other inevitable.

The orthodox religious teaching that stressed the fall of man through the "original sin," and the further indictment that every individual is "conceived in sin," gave a working basis to the theory of mankind's inherent wickedness. So, being steeped in iniquity, it was merely a case of keeping a sharp lookout for it (in everyone else) and exposing the offender whenever possible.

But while this accepted theory of man's depravity presupposed the sinfulness to be inherent, there was always the tendency to associate it in actuality with some extraneous agency—some-

thing apart from his normal human personality.
So, as we have seen, the individual, when found
guilty, was condemned for harbouring within him
some devil or evil spirit, or quality of witchcraft.

In substance, his was a dual character; one human, with all the shortcomings, perhaps, that his
questionable origin assured, but the other positively and irretrievably bad, socially intolerable.
Thus, we can understand the drastic means used
to eliminate the evil—in a blind effort to protect
society—even at the expense of destroying what
may have been tolerably good in the unfortunate
individual.

## Insanity in Retrospect

A more notable instance of the old popular acceptance of dual personality is afforded in the
treatment of the insane.  For ages, up to nearly
the middle of the last century, "crazy" people
were definitely considered to be "possessed" by
various evil spirits.  The insane in many instances
were beaten unmercifully to "drive out" the evil
interlopers, and, when unfortunate enough to survive, were chained in dungeons and otherwise subjected to the most cruel and loathsome treatment.

This conception of insanity, which prevailed
throughout the long period beginning with the
times described in the Old Testament and continu-
ing down through the Middle Ages, has been
termed "demonological."  Insanity was regarded

as the manifestation of some spiritual being who either actually inhabited the body of the subject, or who played upon him from without. In either event, it was supposed to be an extraneous agency at work.

It is interesting to note that among many of the groups, if the phenomena manifested were in harmony with the religious views of the time, it was considered that the controlling spirit was benign in character, and the individual "possessed" was revered as an exceptionally holy person. This explains many of the hallucinatory visions of the Middle Ages when the subjects had discourse with Jesus or the Virgin Mary, and therefore were canonized as saints or recognized as persons enjoying the favour of the Lord.[1]

Among some of the ancients, idiots were thought to be particularly blessed by the gods, and in communion with the heavenly regions. As their actions and talk were not properly understood, it was supposed they were of a supernatural character. It is said that Tycho Brahe, the great astronomer, had an idiot as a constant companion to whose mutterings he listened with profound respect, trusting that he might overhear some

[1] "In the records of the ascetics and ecstatics who flourished at that period, we find manifestations constantly described, visions and trances for example, which are of frequent occurrence in the insane patient of today. The current beliefs of the Middle Ages, however, regarded such phenomena as the result of intimate communion with the Deity, and the individuals in whom they occurred were correspondingly revered and esteemed." Dr. Bernard Hart—*The Psychology of Insanity.*

heavenly communication of astronomic importance.

The vast majority of the persons "possessed," however, came under the category of the baneful type, and were considered to be victims of a malignant devil, which conflicted with the prevailing ethical code.

While science has revolutionized these old conceptions, and we have adopted more rational theories and practices in treating the mentally deranged, we still retain some of the old superstitious feeling in regard to this class of unfortunates. It is true that we do not countenance wilful, studied cruelty in our treatment of the insane, but there is a widespread feeling that in these chaotic, incoherent minds some *foreign,* sinister force is giving vent to itself.

As a result of this general sentiment, we still publicly and officially retain in regard to the insane an attitude of morbid revulsion rather than of humane understanding. Another aspect of this situation is the popular idea of the insane as a separate and distinct class of society—that a vast gulf separates the sane from the insane. As a matter of fact, there are degrees of mental instability and intellectual and emotional vicissitude among those who make up the bulk of the population that fluctuate on an extensive scale, from the very heights of rational conduct right down to the borderline where they cannot readily be discerned from the irresponsible and unbalanced.

*Emotional Appeal of Religion*

This wide overlapping of mental variations, which it is often difficult to define or classify, among the "normal," the neurotic and the insane, is of profound importance and extremely interesting to observe; and it throws a flood of light on the psychic makeup of man. It enables us better to understand some of the duality of his nature and his reactions to his environment. In its proper place, we shall give this subject more adequate consideration.

Perhaps no field of human activity has allowed so much scope for the free functioning of the dual personality as religion. In order to appreciate the significance of this, it is necessary to take into consideration the primitive origin of all the great religions, which had their beginnings in a semi-Oriental setting, at the period of human history when man's attempts at abstract reasoning were largely in terms of mythological concepts.

And the influence of mythology and folklore in the themes of religious literature and the dramatization of its principal episodes and characters is very pronounced. Linked up with this is the great mass of symbolism and mystic ritual which is still retained by the orthodox churches, and which has so strong an appeal to the emotional, as contrasted with the intellectual, side of the personality.

But religion has even a more primitive basis than the theology of the Old and New Testaments, the Koran, the Talmud, Lao Tse's Tao and other sacred writings. Long antedating any written word or existing cipher, the primitive savage and his long line of descendents worshipped at the shrine of Phallus. Realizing his helplessness in a hostile world, surrounded by remorseless enemies and terrifying natural forces whose secrets were not to be revealed until untold centuries later, he sought in his crude, groping way for an Ultimate Cause.

The Caveman in the infancy of the race, therefore, sanctified the functions of his body which gave him the most pleasure, and which reproduced his kind. The generative organs were the obvious physical basis of procreation, the only direct source that he could identify with the origin of life and the continuity of the race, so he venerated that which to him had a tangible connection with Creation. He probably thought it the *source* of Creation.

While Phallicism is now a subject of growing scientific interest, little popular study has been given to it in the past. Nevertheless, it has left its indelible imprint both on the mind of mankind and on the symbolism, ritual and dogma of all the ancient religions that have survived.

The initiated student of today sees the spiritual legacy of our Phallic-worshipping ancestors in some of the finest architecture, ancient and modern, in the world. The Phallus was represented in ancient crosses that were raised in Egypt and other parts of the world centuries before the Christian era. It is symbolized in the pyramids, obelisks and monumental shafts, in steeples and cupolas, in the conventionalized lotus designs, fleur-de-lis and in numerous other forms of ornamentation. The female genitals are symbolized in many varieties of decoration and design, in talismans, charms and in the architecture of churches, cathedrals (as in certain shaped doors, windows and apertures) and other imposing buildings.

Thus we have unconsciously carried down a fast biological heritage and paid our tribute to the Caveman of prehistoric ages. And in so doing we have done the bidding of the Caveman concealed within us today, whose existence is as real as was his unveneered prototype of ages and ages ago.

## BIBLIOGRAPHY

MORGAN, T. H., *A Critique of the Theory of Evolution.* Princeton University Press, 1916.

METCHNIKOFF, E., *The Nature of Man,* Chicago, 1903.

LOEB, J., *The Mechanistic Conception of Life,* Chicago, 1911.

ADAMS, W. H. D., *Witch, Warlock and Magician,* New York, 1889.

HART, BERNARD, *The Psychology of Insanity,* Cambridge University Press, 1920.

MCDOUGALL, WILLIAM, *An Introduction to Social Psychology,* Boston, 1915.

# CHAPTER II

## THE CAVEMAN'S BACKGROUND—OUR PRIMITIVE PERSONALITY

> Out of the past we have come. Into it we are constantly returning. Meanwhile, it is of the utmost importance to our lives. It contains the roots of all we are. . . . It contains the record or ruins of all the experiments that man has made during a quarter or a half million years in the art of living in this world.—CASSIUS J. KEYSER, *Human Worth of Rigorous Thinking.*

A MORE adequate realization of our primitive personality will be gained if we consider for a moment our immeasurably far-reaching biological past. We must take into consideration the lineage we have behind us from primitive man, and for æons before that from prehuman types. There is the basic organism which we have inherited, with its ingrained impressions, instincts and emotions that have been picked up during millions of years of struggle with the remorseless forces of nature. And over the mechanism of this wild and ancient heritage there has been thrown, during the past few thousands of years, a slight coat of cultural whitewash, which may be called the veneer of civilization.

Popularly (and theologically) speaking, man has been in the habit of dating his creation back some 6,000 years, and considering the advent of his prototype as a finished being. This supernatural conception of creation, of course, has been so long exploded by science that it seems almost trite to mention it, and I only do so to emphasize the actual great antiquity of the race, according to estimates of the leading authorities.

### Man's Great Antiquity

Henry Fairfield Osborn says: "The beginning of the Age of Man, some 500,000 years ago, roughly estimated as the close of the Age of Mammals, marks in reality but the beginning of the close of the Age of Mammals. . . . The ascent of man as one of the Primates was parallel with that of the families of apes. Man has a long line of ancestry of his own, *perhaps two million or more years in length.* He is not descended from any *known form* of ape, either living or fossil."

Accepting this hypothesis (which is undoubtedly the best and most authoritative we have), it is impossible for the human imagination to comprehend the real significance of the immense span of time—the millions and millions of years—it took for the evolution of the simplest monocellular structures into and through the metazoa to their present day goal in man.

Biologists are generally agreed that one-celled organisms reached their utmost limits of complexity millions of years ago; since when they have shown many diversities, many adaptations, but little, if any, progress.

Many-celled animals and plants also long ago reached the limits of their possible progress in almost every line. Multiplication of cells, tissues, organs, systems and zooids tremendously increased the possibilities of specialization within the larger units of their organization, but for "millions of years there has been little further progress in this direction of multiplicity and complexity."

In this connection, Professor Conklin remarks that "only about *fourteen times in the whole history of life upon the earth* have new animal phyla appeared, and many of these were mere blind alleys which led nowhere, not even to many species; there have been no new phyla since fishes appeared in the Silurian age, no new classes since mammals appeared in the Triassic and birds in the Jurassic."[1]

The earliest type of man-like creature so far discovered is the erect ape-man, *Pithecanthropus erectus,* the remains of which were found in Trinil, Java, by Dubois in 1892. These fossils were found in a geological formation which included many ex-

[1] Edwin Grant Conklin, *The Direction of Human Evolution,* Scribner's, 1921.

tinct mammals of the late Pliocene or pre-glacial period, estimated at 500,000 years ago.

Even a half million years ago, the human line was already distinct from the higher apes, although much closer than at present. The period at which they came together is assumed to be a million or a million and a half years earlier.[2]

Skeletal remains have been found which indicate, in connection with stratigraphical evidences,

[2] "But man is not simply a 'developed ape.' Apes and men have diverged from the same primitive stock—apelike, manlike, but not exactly one nor the other. No apes nor monkeys now extant could apparently have been ancestors of primitive man. None could ever 'develop' into man. As man changes and diverges, race into race, so do they. The influence of effort, the influence of surroundings, the influence of the sifting process of natural selection, each acts upon them as it acts upon man. The process of evolution is not progress, but better adaptation to conditions of life. As man becomes fitted for social and civic life, so does the ape become fitted for life in the tree-tops. The movement of monkeys is toward simianity, not humanity. The movement of cat life is toward felinity, that of the dog races toward caninity. Each step in evolution upward or downward, whatever it may be, carries each species or type farther from the primitive stock. These steps are never retraced. For an ape to become a man he must go back to the simple characters of the simple common type from which both have sprung. These characters are shown in the ape baby and in the human embryo in its corresponding stages, for ancestral traits lost in the adult are evident in the young. This persistence comes through the operation of the great force of cell memory which we call heredity. The evidence of biology points to the descent of all mammals, of all vertebrates, of all animals, of all organic beings, from a common stock. Of all the races of animals the anthropoid apes are the nearest to man. Their divergence from the same stock must be comparatively recent. Man is the nomadic, the apes are the arboreal, branch of the same great family." David Starr Jordan—*Footnotes to Evolution.*

that in Europe the existing species of man (Homo-sapiens) goes back at least 20,000 to 30,000 years.

These few but impressive biological hypotheses are cited chiefly to bring to attention the long primitive heritage of the race, which will better enable us to comprehend the basically primitive nature of the individual.

### Inherent Prehuman Modes of Action

Man, according to the specific theory of John Dewey, and in substance to that of E. L. Thorndike, is a mosaic of original, *ineradicable, and unlearned tendencies to action,* an equipment of behavior-unit characters. The several paragraphs preceding roughly indicate the process whereby man acquired this ineradicable mosaic character.

The best way to understand the dynamic influence of these biological traits is to begin with the new-born child, and observe its course through infancy, childhood, adolescence to mature adulthood.

The late Carleton Parker remarked that he looked on with astonishment, mixed with conventional moral indignation, when Prof. John B. Watson forced an hour-old, wailing American infant to swing seven minutes by its one-handed grip on a lead pencil. A negro baby with a more recent and virile biological memory swung fourteen minutes.[3]

Indeed, the clinging instinct is one of the most potent of the reflex modes of response of the infant. It is a defensive equipment, having its origin in the necessity of the prehuman ape-baby clinging to the shaggy hair of its mother who ranged among the trees, and later developed by its own tree ranging. The hands of the young baby never remain wide open. The flexor muscles of the fingers are always in a state of contraction. They attempt to grasp everything they can lay their hands on, and if there is nothing within reach for them to cling to, they keep their hands closed tightly in imitation of the act of holding on. This characteristic of the primates is an acquirement of the arboreal past. Alfred Russel Wallace once caught a young monkey and as he was carrying it home in his arms the little simian fingers happened to come in contact with the naturalist's whiskers, and held on so tightly that he had great difficulty in getting them loose.

The human baby, as we have seen, has remarkable development of the forearm muscles at birth, possessing in this respect much greater relative strength than the average adult, notwithstanding the constant exercise of the arm muscles throughout the active period of life. And nothing gives the baby so much pleasure as to get its little fingers tangled up in somebody's hair.

[3] Carleton H. Parker, *The Casual Labourer and Other Essays.*

Contrast the muscular development of the new-born infant's arm with that of any other part of the body—the legs, for instance. The muscles of the body, legs and neck require many months of development before they can perform even for brief periods the duties eventually dependent upon them, whereas the muscles of the infant's arm and hand, at birth, will usually enable it to sustain the entire weight of its body for a period of from a few seconds to several minutes. This is, indeed, a remarkable feat that requires some explanation —and only the biological heritage of the individual, with its survival of primitive instincts, offers a satisfactory explanation.

It has been said that the child is a born savage. It is even worse than that. At birth, human beings are quadrupeds. Their earliest attempts at locomotion are on all-fours. The natural position of the thighs is at right angles with the general position of the body, as in other quadrupeds. Observe a young baby lying on its back and free to assume a natural position of the limbs. The legs do not extend straight out, as in adults. They stick straight up, as in a four-legged animal.

### Law of Recapitulation

Now let us trace the primitive characteristics of the individual back through much earlier stages. We shall use as our guide the Law of

Recapitulation, or the Law of Biogenesis, as it is sometimes called. The Biogenetic Law means a certain uniformity which exists from the beginning of life, namely: *"Every organism in its development repeats the life history of the race to which it belongs."* For example, every reptile is a fish before it is a reptile; every bird is a fish before it is a bird; every mammal is a fish before it is a mammal.

There is a time in the embryonic development of all higher vertebrates when they have not only a fish shape but breathe by gills like fishes and have two chambered hearts and the peculiar circulation of the fish. Whereas fishes have two-chambered hearts, frogs have three-chambered hearts; reptiles have hearts with three chambers and the beginning of a fourth; and birds and mammals have complete four-chambered hearts.

A bird or mammal does not develop a four-chambered heart the first thing. The beginning of the circulatory system of a bird or mammal is a pulsating tube, as in a worm. Later it acquires a two-chambered heart, like the fish, then a three-chambered heart, like the frog, then the beginning of four chambers, like the reptile, and finally the complete four-chambered heart of its race.

The following tabulation shows the chief classes of the animal kingdom as they exist on the earth today. This classification is arranged roughly in the order from the lowest to the highest, the lowest being at the bottom:

CLASSES OF ANIMALS

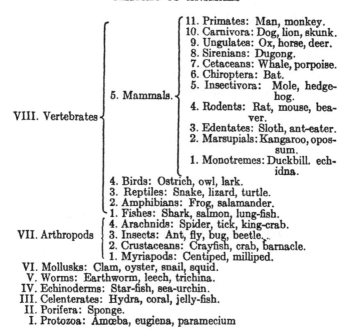

VIII. Vertebrates

5. Mammals.
11. Primates: Man, monkey.
10. Carnivora: Dog, lion, skunk.
9. Ungulates: Ox, horse, deer.
8. Sirenians: Dugong.
7. Cetaceans: Whale, porpoise.
6. Chiroptera: Bat.
5. Insectivora: Mole, hedge-hog.
4. Rodents: Rat, mouse, bea-ver.
3. Edentates: Sloth, ant-eater.
2. Marsupials: Kangaroo, opos-sum.
1. Monotremes: Duckbill. ech-idna.

4. Birds: Ostrich, owl, lark.
3. Reptiles: Snake, lizard, turtle.
2. Amphibians: Frog, salamander.
1. Fishes: Shark, salmon, lung-fish.

VII. Arthropods
4. Arachnids: Spider, tick, king-crab.
3. Insects: Ant, fly, bug, beetle.
2. Crustaceans: Crayfish, crab, barnacle.
1. Myriapods: Centiped, milliped.

VI. Mollusks: Clam, oyster, snail, squid.
V. Worms: Earthworm, leech, trichina.
IV. Echinoderms: Star-fish, sea-urchin.
III. Celenterates: Hydra, coral, jelly-fish.
II. Porifera: Sponge.
I. Protozoa: Amœba, eugiena, paramecium

Geologists have noted that there are no remains of back-boned animals in the lowest rocks. The oldest fossil cemeteries of the earth are filled entirely with invertebrates, because away back in that remote period of our planet when these ancient burying grounds were being filled, there were no back-boned animals in existence.

Science teaches us that the first inhabitants of this world were those whose names stand at the bottom of the foregoing list—the protozoa. *Zoa* is the Greek word for "animals," and *protos* means "first"—thus *Protozoa* means the "first animals"; therefore the common ancestors of all other animals. All other creatures have developed directly or indirectly from these primordial ancestors of animal life on this globe.

Every animal goes through a series of changes or processes of evolution before arriving at maturity. Regardless of whether it is a clam, a beetle, or a frog, an elephant or a man, it always begins as a one-celled animal—or protozoan—a microscopic speck. We all go back to the beginning of life.

In the developing embryo of the vertebrate—to pass over the lower orders—which begins with the protozoan, it will eventually get a series of bones extending along the back through which runs a nerve-cord with an enlargement at the front end called the brain. It will also develop a heart of two chambers and the peculiar circulation of the fish, and breathe with gills.

In the case of the frog, it will finally abandon its gills as breathing organs, and get lungs, and legs and a three-chambered heart. If it is a bird or mammal, it will develop a four-chambered heart, either feathers, fur or hair, as the case may be, and the characteristic form of its species.

There is, however, always a stage in the embryonic development of birds and mammals when they breathe with gills like a fish and have other general characteristics of the fish. Human beings have been born with gill-slits open in the neck. The human embryo is surrounded by a watery substance, the *amniotic fluid*. The fishes were the pioneer vertebrates, and all other vertebrates have evolved from them, and so all the higher vertebrates as individuals pass through the fish stage in fulfilment of the biogenetic law.

Of course, it is understood that because of the rapid prenatal development of the individual— which in the case of the human being evolves from the microscopic, fertilized ovum to the completely formed baby in nine months—the stages are not clearly defined nor distinct. The individual in a few months passes through changes that have taken the race millions of years to undergo. A hundred million years may be as good a guess as any. The individual development, is, therefore, not a detailed recapitulation of the racial development, but an outline or synopsis with the various stages largely fused and indistinct. But notwithstanding the omissions and modifications, the biogenetic law remains as one of the most remarkable truths in the whole range of biology.

⁴Man, and all the mammals, still carry the birthmarks of their common ancestry from the fish, the amphibian and reptilian species. A chicken of three or four days' incubation has four gill-slits on the side of its neck. In human embryos of three to five weeks' development, these gill-slits appear. All reptiles, birds and mammals possess them. They serve no function with purely air-breathing creatures, and, except in rare instances, close long before hatching or birth. In the early embryos of all higher forms of life is found the notachord—the dorsal stiffening axis of the lower vertebrates. This disappears as the backbone develops.

Biologists rely on this law to a great extent in tracing the relationships of animals. For instance, the members of two different species of animals may, as adults, look very much alike and may seem to be closely akin. But if it is found that they differ widely in their individual development, that is, as individuals go through widely different series of embryonic changes—they are likely to be put into entirely different categories.

The development of the race from animal ancestry seems to be particularly distressing to the religious and philosophic belief of many people. There should be no more shock felt over this hypothesis of the origin of the race, than over the fact that the individual has a germinal origin. This latter phenomenon is so self-evident that it cannot be questioned. And yet, the belief in a supernaturally created human being is on a par with the "stork" explanation of the individual's birth.

### Mental Recapitulation

The same parallelism that exists between the physical evolution of the individual and the race, exists between the *mental* development of the individual and the race.

In all mammals, including man, the brain at one stage of development is like that of a fish. And just as the brain of the higher animals, including man, has been built up step by step through a process of evolution extending back millions of years into the past, so has the mind of man likewise developed step by step through an evolutionary process extending back millions of years into the past.

The new-born baby cannot think. But the continuance of its existence is made possible by a few powerful instincts, primarily the urge to suck (thereby obtaining nourishment); the defensive tendency to cling (a vestigial desire to adhere to the body of its mother); and the craving to escape the annoying reality of its new world through sleep, (symbolizing possibly a return to the uniform warmth and comfort of its prenatal existence, where every want was automatically cared for and no desire left unfulfilled). The biochemical memories of the prenatal state are strong in adulthood also, and a symbolized return to this condition of supreme satisfaction has been universally noted, as we shall evidence later.

Born deaf and blind, the infant soon begins to see, hear, taste, and feel more pronouncedly pain and satisfaction. At about three weeks, the basic emotions begin to manifest themselves. The first emotions a child has are those of fear and surprise. Before we have the power to love or hate or comprehend, we are *able to be afraid*. This conforms to the defensive reactions of mankind's remote prehuman ancestors, who were protected by this prompting to fear and flee from ever-alert enemies.

At the age of ten weeks, curiosity and pugnacity show themselves. It is perhaps natural that the tendency to fight should follow so closely the disposition to flee. At twelve weeks, jealousy and anger and exhibitions of the play instinct usually appear, and the mind begins to perform the most elementary acts of mental association, as, for instance, associating the sight of a bottle with food.

At fourteen weeks, reason and affection begin to dawn, vaguely to be sure. Sympathy and the desire to express ideas appear at about the age of five months. Pride, resentment and appreciation of pleasing objects begin to assert themselves at eight months; grief, hate and cruelty at ten months; revenge and tool-using at twelve months; and shame, remorse and deceit at fifteen months.

There is a striking resemblance between the evolution of the child's mind from birth to about the age of one or one and one-half years, and the evolution of mind in the animal kingdom up to the advent of man.

Beginning with the age of one or one and one-half years, the mind of the civilized child is an outline, crude but unmistakable, of the prehistoric evolution of the human race. The child is a savage, with the emotional reactions peculiar to savages; with the conceptions of the world common among savages; and with the desires, pastimes and ambitions of the savage. What young boy does not envy the life of the American Indian? The male Indian did practically no confining work. The females baked the pottery, wove the blankets, cultivated the maize, and performed the drudgery and routine duties. The stalwart brave hunted, fished, smoked his pipe, and occasionally went on the warpath. These are all primitive pastimes, and all of them still fulfil the rôle of an emotional outlet for the primitive cravings of modern man. Children are dominated by these primitive emotions; normal adult persons, who have succeeded in adapting themselves to their social environment, have learned to conform, more or less, to certain general requirements of our civilization; but within every individual, under this surface conformity, there remains intact all the old mechanism of the primitive savage. The manifold operations of this mechanism, along its old primal paths, will be discussed in detail later.

Lying, or rather unintentional disregard for the truth, and other ethical shortcomings, judged by the best cultural standards, are characteristic of the young child, as they are of the savage. Even at the present day, travelers remark how prone the savage is to forgetfulness; how, after a short tension of memory, his mind begins to sway here and there from sheer weariness and gives forth lies and foolishness.

Every infant likes to wield a stick or similar object, with which it bangs away right and left. This is reminiscent of the club-using period. The Big Stick was the first weapon—a ready means of defense and offense.

The youth covets a jackknife like no other toy. There are indelible biological memories, resulting in an instinctive attraction, connected with the knife. For a long, long time in the infancy of the race, the knife meant food and life. With it, man battled with his enemies and secured his sustenance. Other primitive weapons were the sling and the bow and arrow. Man's fondness for whittling as a diversion has the same origin as his fondness for hunting, fishing, fighting and the rivalry of sports.

The development of childhood is a rapid recapitulation of the successive emotional stages of evolving mankind. It is important for the development of the fullest possibilities of the child that this fact should be understood. These emotional cravings of childhood should neither be denied nor thwarted—but should be *directed,* and an appropriate outlet assured for each progressive stage of the evolving individual. If the basic emotions are suppressed or repressed, the mind, unconsciously for the most part, will, in adult years, seek to return to its cheated childhood in a symbolical form. The vital significance of this proposition will be discussed more fully in a subsequent chapter.

Adolescence is perhaps the crucial period in the life of the youth. It is the turning point—from childhood to adulthood. It involves the large emotional urges signifying the rounding out of childhood (corresponding to the transition stage from barbarism to civilization in the evolution of the race) and the innovation of new physiological factors, with their far-reaching psychological reactions.

It is at this important period that the habits formed through childhood are hardened into the inflexible mould that is destined to shape well nigh irretrievably the individual's future. The many influences of environment, so important at all times, are vital at this period. This situation led the late Professor Lester Ward to call the skilful and daring criminal "the genius of the slums." By this expressive term, which is a sad commentary on the irrational structure of our social organization, it is meant that when native talent or genius finds its birthright cheated by the blight of the slums, its course too often becomes perverted through the sordid surroundings and lack of constructive opportunity. And in order to satisfy the craving for excitement and achievement, to secure an outlet for the expression of the powerful ego urge, it almost inevitably develops along some anti-social channel—into the adroit crook, or master-criminal.

### *Autonomic Nervous System*

Our primitive personality could hardly be discussed without, at least, some passing reference to the autonomic nervous system, and the endocrine or ductless glands. These are the automatic working bases of the animal organism that so strongly attract the attention both of the modern physiologists and psychologists.

The biological history which we have briefly summarized indicates the way our organism has developed, and emphasizes its primitive *past*. A study of the nervous system and ductless glands demonstrates the development as it *is,* and permits us to look into the operation of our basic personality—our primitive *present.*

Intelligence, intellect and cultural development are possible only with a finely organized, balanced nervous system. A crude, unstable nervous system precludes unusual or even ordinary development of these qualities. Dr. Smith Ely Jelliffe has said: "Bones, tendons, muscles, intestines, hearts, lungs, have been much alike for countless centuries, and have modified little in their structure, but the nervous system, an active, changing master-spirit in evolution, is constantly reaching out in its attempt to grasp the infinite."

But notwithstanding its higher qualities and potentialities, the nervous system is inherently and inescapably primitive. It is true that it can be trained, cultivated or sublimated to an extent —sometimes to a very great extent—but essentially and basically, it harkens to the memories of the millions of years behind it. The call of the past is too deeply rooted and too real to be overcome or ignored. Normally or abnormally, it will assert itself. It is a wise person who knows the nature of this old troglodyte that can be influenced to a measureable extent only by the ethical and cultural factors of civilization.

Both the normal and abnormal manifestations of the primitive personality will be covered at length in other chapters. For the present, we will consider merely some of the normal operations of the autonomic nervous system, and the glands through which it makes itself felt so effectively.

The autonomic nervous system is the defensive signal service and operating agency of the body that permits the organism to exist. It is safe to say that the human body as constructed, with all its vulnerable spots, surrounded with such hazards as prevail in the every-day world, could not exist without the elaborate nervous system, or some similar arrangement, that has developed with the anatomy.

Every move of the autonomic system (which controls the involuntary muscles, the heart beats, the respiration, the digestive and excretory organs, the contraction or enlargement of the pupil of the eye, regulates the sweat glands, and performs manifold other operations) has a defensive object—a self or racial preservation motive. Its original response for millions of years was limited to self-preservation through the defensive medium of instant preparation for flight or fight; stimulating the desire for subsistence and pleasure through the appetite; and assuring race preservation through the channels of the reproductive in-

stinct (which is also an appetite or urge). Hence
we have today the vital force of these factors
which operates either undisguised, as it sometimes
does to an extent; or modified and symbolized, as
it is in many ways, to conform to the changed
conditions of modern society.

All the numerous organs and glands of the body
are regulated by the autonomic nervous system.
And there is always the definite motive of fostering agreeable appetites, leading to the upkeep of
the individual and the continuance of the race;
or of instigating a means of defense—through
fright, flight or fight. Now the conditions favorable to these two general categories of action are
invariably opposed. When we are in a condition
favorable for the appeasement of the appetite for
food, we are not prepared for flight or fight. And,
as it is well known, when we are frightened or
grieved, we are in no condition to take or digest
food.

Therefore, the autonomic nervous system plays
a dual rôle: (1) As an agency of defense and offense for the protection of the individual, through
the functioning of the sympathetic division; and
(2), As an agency contributing to the immediate
comfort and pleasure of the individual, through
the operation of the vagotonic division (consti-
tuting the cranial and sacral sections). Thus,
when we feel disposed to enjoy a good meal, the
cranial section of the autonomic system causes the
saliva in the mouth and the gastric juices in the

stomach to flow freely. If some danger should suddenly impend, the sympathetic division checks these digestive activities (our mouth becomes dry, and the stomach undergoes a similar change) so that we have neither the desire, nor, to an extent, the ability to eat. The danger signal has been raised by an *automatic action within us* (which is not subject to our conscious control, although intelligence enables us sometimes to modify the action in a measure). The meaning of this is that the paramount urge of self-protection has become operative. If it is a false alarm, the effect is no less real while it lasts. The efficiency of this nervous organization has contributed to the preservation of individual life and the perpetuation of the species during the millions of years that this nervous system has been developing and perfecting itself.

The opposing activities of the two divisions of this nervous organization will be observed in the following manifestations: The sympathetic dilates the pupil of the eye (a characteristic of fear), while the cranial contracts it (signifying contentment and well-being); the sympathetic accelerates the action of the heart (enabling it to respond to greater physical demands, primitively for defensive struggle), while the cranial slows it down (giving it longer periods of rest); the sympathetic relaxes the lower part of the large intestine (freeing the body of an incumbrance to flight), while the sacral contracts it, and so on.

### The Ductless Glands

There are certain accessories to the defensive nerve mechanism of the body that deserve brief mention. Prominent of these are the adrenals and other ductless glands, like the thyroid, parathyroid, pineal, thymus and pituitary glands, for instance, which produce internal secretions that act upon the body directly through the blood. The adrenals are small glands lying anterior to each kidney. Their secretion, adrenin, when infused into the blood causes the pupils to dilate, hairs to stand erect, the activities of the alimentary canal to be inhibited, blood vessels to be constricted, and sugar to be liberated from the liver. The adrenal glands are therefore very important defensive units of the organism, and l ve a deep bearing on the emotions of the individual. In other words, they are *vital elements of the primitive personality.*

It was once thought the emotions were psychic manifestations exclusively. Now we know that they are largely physiological, and always have a physical basis. Emotions, attitudes and secretions ever go together. It is impossible to experience one without the other two. A secretion will produce an emotion, and an emotion will produce an attitude or "state of mind." An attitude will produce an appropriate secretion, which in turn will result in an emotion. An emotion must have the physiological basis of a secretion or there would be no quickening of the pulse, no rising of color in the face, no arousing of the physical being generally—no thrill; in substance, no emotion.

Adrenin also reinforces the sympathetic impulses in other ways than noted—all lending to the protection of the individual.  It restores a tired or fatigued muscle or organ to its original ability after being subjected to activity through a prolonged period.  This explains the phenomenon of "second wind" which enables the tired athlete to continue with even better results, after the first feeling of overpowering fatigue.  William James (*The Energies of Man*) suggested that in every person there are "reservoirs of power" which are not ordinarily called upon, but which are nevertheless ready to pour forth streams of energy whenever the occasion demands it.  The functions of the body we are discussing give us an inkling as to the source of this power.

Another preservative influence of adrenin on the body is its value as a coagulating agency.  If a person is wounded while in a passion (as in fighting), that is, when there is a maximum of adrenin and glycogen (sugar) in the blood, the latter will coagulate much more rapidly than if he is wounded while emotionally composed.

And the major emotions—fear, rage, pain, the pangs of hunger, etc.—are shared alike by man and beast.  Similar tests under similar conditions will produce similar results in man and the higher animals.

The body in the stress of exertion, pain and strong emotional excitement calls upon the liver for the supply of glycogen or sugar; this is the form in which carbohydrate material is transported in the organisms. Starch is the storage form. When needed, this reserve supply is liberated in the blood in the form of sugar. In the bodies of well-fed animals, the liver contains an abundance of glycogen or "animal starch," which is potential blood sugar.

It has been noted that prolonged grief or anxiety in a great crisis so increases the sugar in the blood that acute, and sometime chronic diabetes results. A medical writer cites the case of a German officer whose diabetes and Iron Cross for valour both came from a hazardous experience in the Franco-Prussian War.

In repeated experimentation on cats, dogs, rabbits and other animals, copious increases of sugar in the blood were noted after the animals had been excited or enraged. Urine tests before and after the experiment clearly indicated the accuracy of the reaction.

Professor Cannon[5] reports a test wherein four of nine medical students, all normally without sugar in their urine, had glycosuria after a hard examination, and only one of the nine had gly-

[5] Walter B. Cannon, *Bodily Changes in Pain, Hunger, Fear and Rage.*

cosuria after an easier examination. A study was made on second-year students at a woman's college. Of thirty-six who had no sugar in the urine on the day before, six, or seventeen per cent., eliminated sugar with the urine passed immediately after examination.

Twenty-five members of the Harvard University football squad were examined immediately after the final and most exciting contest one season and sugar was found in twelve cases. Five of these positive cases were among substitutes not called upon to enter the game. Nevertheless, they were under intense emotional excitement. The only excited spectator of the Harvard victory whose urine was examined also had a marked glycosuria, which on the following day had disappeared.

The pituitary gland, which lies in a bony setting at the base of the brain, behind the root of the nose, governs the growth of the skeleton, muscles, ligaments and tendons, influences the sexual processes and assists in energy transformation, energy expenditure and conversion. It is the gland of continued effort.

The thyroid, located in the neck, astride the windpipe, also has a fundamental bearing on the growth and development of body and mind. This is demonstrated in the instance of persons suffering from subnormal action of the thyroid. If severe, the skin becomes dry and rough, peeling in sheets. The hair becomes shaggy and coarse, like an animal's; the temperature drops to a subnormal point. All ambition disappears and the subject becomes apathetic, indifferent, awkward, even approaching some degree of idiocy.

The remarkable feature about this is, if the victim is given thyroxin (the secretion of the thyroid gland) he is soon transformed in all his physical and mental qualities, and remains so as long as the treatment is consistently continued. The skin, the hair, the temperature, and the mental processes all become normal, or relatively so.

The other ductless glands, although less spectacular in their functions, are vitally important, but space will not permit discussing them.

The chief value in citing the foregoing physiological factors and tests is to illustrate our physical kinship with the animal world, and thereby emphasize the primitive *basis* of our emotions, which constitute the unconscious or spontaneous *expression of our personality*. As it has been stated, we have been in the habit of attributing to mental effort many of our actions which are purely reflexes of physiological origin. They are the defensive mechanism of our primitive personality.

A great many ''states of mind'' or attitudes are due to causes predisposed by our physical constitution. They are simply reactions of the autonomic nervous system—which has a longer biological development than the sensori-motor nervous system—and over which we have no direct control. As adults, our indirect control over the functions of the autonomic system is limited to the moderate (but in effect, relatively great) extent that we are able to influence them by a rational outlook on life, which presupposes a rational insight into our real nature. And the prime object of this book is to help in disseminating this knowledge, so essential to a healthy, well-balanced life.

### BIBLIOGRAPHY

OSBORN, HENRY FAIRFIELD, *Men of the Old Stone Age,* New York.

OSBORN, HENRY FAIRFIELD, *The Origin and Evolution of Life,* New York.

CONKLIN, EDWIN GRANT, *The Direction of Human Evolution,* New York, 1921.

WATSON, JOHN B., *Psychology from the Standpoint of a Behaviorist,* Philadelphia, 1919.

JORDAN, DAVID STARR, *Footnotes to Evolution,* New York.

MOORE, J. HOWARD, *The Law of Biogenesis,* Chicago, 1914.

MOORE, J. HOWARD, *Savage Survivals,* Chicago, 1916.

CANNON, WALTER B., *Bodily Changes in Pain, Hunger, Fear and Rage,* New York, 1920.

CRILE, G. W., *The Origin and Nature of the Emotions,* Philadelphia, 1915.

CRILE, G. W., *Man, an Adaptive Mechanism,* New York, 1916.

DARWIN, CHARLES, *Origin of Species.*

DARWIN, CHARLES, *Descent of Man.*

DRIESCH, H., *The Science and Philosophy of the Organism,* London, 1908.

LOEB, JACQUES, *The Organism as a Whole—from a Physico-chemical Viewpoint,* New York, 1915.

BOAS, FRANZ, *The Mind of Primitive Man*, New York, 1921.

LAVASTINE, M. L., *The Internal Secretions and the Nervous System*, New York.

MORGAN, T. H., *The Physical Basis of Heredity*, Philadelphia.

GALTON, FRANCIS, *Natural Inheritance*, London, 1889.

SPENCER, HERBERT, *Principles of Biology*, New York, 1883.

BERMAN, LOUIS, *Glands Regulating the Personality*, New York, 1921.

HARROW, BENJAMIN, *Glands in Health and Disease*, New York, 1922.

CHAPTER III

## THE CAVEMAN'S VENEER—OUR CULTURAL PERSONALITY AND ITS POSSIBILITIES

*The man of prehistoric times lives on, unchanged, in our Unconscious.*—SIGMUND FREUD.

WHILE the cultural side of the personality has received more attention than the primitive, which we have just reviewed, the popular conception of it has been very much romanticized. Indeed, by virtually ignoring our early biological background, it was impossible to get a true perspective of the surface strata of our nature which alone has been exposed to social development. The importance of mankind's mass intelligence and culture has been greatly over-emphasized.

It is true that much has been accomplished in the few thousands of years that are recorded in human history. The greater part of human progress, however, is due to a more or less mechanical acceleration of social forces, fostered by the broad economic motive. Progress that is influenced by technology and positive sciences tends to increase geometrically.[1] The advance in

[1] "It ust be admitted that to a considerable extent the progress thus procured has been only technical; it has provided more efficient means for satisfying pre-existent desires rather than modi-

civilization has meant, primarily, only improvement in environment; whereas, neither environment nor training seems to have changed perceptibly the hereditary capabilities of man. Aside from this, an honest review of mankind's activities, since the dawn of history, suggests a none too reassuring picture of a very archaic force blindly cutting its way to an indefinite objective in the destructive manner of a huge cosmic Juggernaut.

The actions of man in his personal and social, and national and international, relations are, broadly speaking, irrational, paradoxical and highly suggestive of the stage of prehistoric savagery through which he has passed. This refers not only to the actual physical combat, treachery, cruelty, vindictiveness and other evidences of a primitive nature, but also to the prevalence of deceit, cunning, lies, bluster, and the like, which are so universal: witness any phase of our social organization—international diplomacy, typical tendencies of newspapers, politics, and other paramount modern influences which need no further comment.

Every great cultural achievement or truly social advance can be matched by many examples of

fied the quality of human purposes. There is, for example, no modern civilization which is the equal of Greek culture in all respects. Science is still too recent to have been absorbed into imaginative and emotional disposition. Men move more swiftly and surely to the realization of their ends, but their ends too largely remain what they were prior to scientific enlightenment.''
—John Dewey.

atavistic destructiveness and continuous practices antagonistic to the common weal. Man is a paradox because of the primitive emotions he feels and the visions he sees. Man, collectively, presents a greater paradox because in his group relations he more quickly reverts to the emotional status of the primitive hunting pack, and sinks to a lower biological level than the individual is apt to do. And, collectively, institutionally, he brags of his culture (or "kultur," depending upon geographical boundaries), democracy, philanthropy, and other cherished national virtues that are as transparent as is his individual veneer of civilization.

The redeeming feature of this has been the few luminous lights, here and there, rising in protest against the unbridled folly, pointing the way to a saner course, and a higher goal. These exceptional people have not been held back by the Caveman within them, chained to one of his primitive levels, but have used his vital, motivating energy to advance a worthy ideal.

There is indeed a cultural personality, and mankind has a cultural history. And notwithstanding the prevailing notion, we of the twentieth century have not a monopoly of its quality. Just as the past decade has brought to the surface some of the worst phases of human nature, has shown us in innumerable cases the Caveman in his wildest excesses, so we can look back, century after century, and see evidences—somewhat isolated, perhaps—of personal culture, mental vigour, and intellectual achievement, that cannot be excelled today. A sweeping statement, you may say, but let us see. After all, what are the four, five and six thousand years of which we have record, in comparison with the untold ages during which man and his predecessors were evolving?

### Early Culture

Let us look into the background of our culture, and compare the *quality* of it today with that of some hundreds, or a couple of thousands of years ago. In quantity, such as it is, there is no comparison, because knowledge (but not intellectual capacity) has increased like the proverbial snowball rolled over a carpet of soft, adhesive snow, collecting layer upon layer as long as the process is continued. The experiences of past generations have been handed down, each succeeding generation adding little or much to the wealth of knowledge that has been bequeathed to it, although never approaching the real possibilities that lie dormant therein. The potentialities are accumulating, but their constructive utilization is relatively subordinated to that of a destructive or dubious character.

As a casual illustration of destructive versus constructive tendencies in our social organization at present, we might compare the national resources used for war purposes (i.e., paying debts incurred in past wars and making preparation for future wars) with those for education, which is conceded to be the basis of our national culture and progress. The actual expenditures of the United States during the fiscal year 1919-1920, for education, research, public health and development, amounted to fifty-nine million dollars, while the expenses for the same period, incident to war, amounted to 3238 millions.[2] Fifty-five times more of the public funds were used in behalf of the destructive caprices of the Caveman, and in catering to his instincts, than for purposes of education and of adding to our cultural possibilities.

A diagrammatic illustration might enable us better to understand the powerful urge behind these atavistic tendencies. That these tendencies exist and must be taken into account is a fact that can be faced with some degree of optimism. When a person becomes aware of why he acts instinctively in a stereotyped way, in certain situations, or reacts in an irrational manner to certain stimuli, he will be more apt to modify his actions to conform to a higher level of social ethics, as he does in many concrete, practical ways. The fanatic who shouts "fire" in a crowded hall is dealt with severely, and means are taken to handle the situation rationally when a fire does occur under similar circumstances. But all over the country—and the world—all kinds of alarmists are virtually shouting "fire" whenever it serves

[2] See *The Next War*, by Will Irwin.

their own purpose. As it is unquestionably impossible to silence these alarmists without at the same time stifling expression of opinion generally, a widespread knowledge of some of the fundamentals of the psychology of behavior would accomplish a beneficial result. To recur to the concrete illustration we have used, extensive publicity and popular propaganda have taught great masses of people something of their psychology in relation to fire in a crowded building. And this knowledge, plus the precautions of exits, maybe the presence of a fireman and a few practical rules of conduct, have prevented many panics. However, all these precautions, without the primary psychological insight would hardly avert a panic in a crisis.

The distressing factor is that the anti-social, destructive proclivities are so often idealized, glorified and fostered, instead of immunizing ourselves against them by a scientific understanding of their nature.

In the previous chapter, I have referred to the great biological heritage of man. The physical and the psychic are so completely interrelated that both are affected by any emotional stimulus. If the major emotions—fear, rage, hate, love, etc. —are recognized as psychic phenomena, they have a physical basis in the functions of the autonomic nervous system and the secretions of the endocrine glands. Every alarmist consciously or unconsciously panders to the more primitive of these emotions (fear, rage, hate), and we can look around at the world for some indication of the result. The "ghosts of the past" too often return to mock our vaunted civilization. They return so readily because they are only under the skin—always with us, ready to stalk across our path.

The diagrammatic suggestion on this page is, of course, purely an arbitrary arrangement, designed

THE HERITAGE OF THE PAST THAT INFLUENCES OUR PRESENT

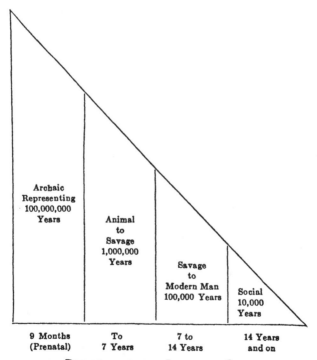

Archaic
Representing
100,000,000
Years

Animal
to
Savage
1,000,000
Years

Savage
to
Modern Man
100,000 Years

Social
10,000
Years

| 9 Months (Prenatal) | To 7 Years | 7 to 14 Years | 14 Years and on |

RECAPITULATION OF INDIVIDUAL LIFE

merely to convey a general idea, as the development of the individual represents a rapid fusing and much overlapping of the evolutionary stages in the recapitulation sense. This diagram, while by no means showing the true proportions, tends to emphasize the tremendous influence of the past over the present, and a great deal of this past we live over today, in a more or less distorted, symbolical form. It also impresses upon us that while the higher social and cultural development of man is relatively new, it is nevertheless a fact that can be made the most of only by a working knowledge of the total situation.

### Intellectual Capacity and Knowledge

While obviously knowledge is becoming more widespread, let us consider the comparative intellectual capacity of man during the past few thousands of years. Are there any minds of today that excel those of Socrates, Aristides, Aristotle and some of their contemporaries? The evidence seems to prove that there has been no perceptible improvement, either physically or in intellectual capacity, in the human race within historic times. The physical beauty of the long-forgotten individuals who posed for the ancient Grecian and Roman statuary is the marvel of all art lovers. And these early models, immortalized in stone and bronze, have become accepted as standards of human anatomical perfection, no less than the sculpturing has as examples of classic artistic production.

And as far as the intellectual side of it goes, the foremost authorities on anthropology, heredity and eugenics maintain that no modern race of men is the intellectual equal of the ancient Greek race.

Sir Francis Galton, the father of eugenics, has called our attention to the fact that in the century between 530 and 430 B.C., in the small country of Attica, there were produced fourteen illustrious men, one for every 4300 of the free-born, adult male population. In the two centuries from 500 to 300 B.C., this small country, about the same size and with a total population equal to that of the state of Rhode Island, but with less than twenty per cent. as many free persons, produced over two dozen illustrious men, whose achievements are enduring in time. The philosophers and men of science included Socrates, Aristotle, Plato, Demetrius and Theophrastus; orators, Demosthenes, Lysias, Æschines and Isocrates; statesmen and commanders, Aristides, Themistocles, Pericles, Cimon, Phocion and Miltiades; poets and dramatists, Sophocles, Euripides, Aristophanes, and Æschylus; artists and architects, Phidias, Polygnotus, Ictinus and Praxiteles; historians Xenophon and Thucydides.

Galton concludes that the average ability of the Athenian race of that period was, on the lowest estimate, as much greater than that of the Anglo-

Saxon race of the present date as the latter is above that of the African negro. It is his opinion that if the Athenians had maintained their excellence and had multiplied and spread over large countries, displacing inferior populations (which they might well have done, for they were naturally very prolific), "they would assuredly have accomplished results advantageous to human civilization to a degree that transcends our powers of imagination." He attributes the decline of this marvelously developed race to a disintegrating state of social morality, which led to promiscuous interbreeding with inferior peoples.

It is interesting in this connection to consider Bateson's suggestion that the high intellectual qualities of the ancient Greeks were due to the inbreeding of homogeneous and very superior phratries and gentes, but that when marriage with aliens was sanctioned, the population gradually mongrelized and its intellectual superiority declined. Vernon Kellogg favors inbreeding as the surest way of preserving the good qualities of a race. William McDougall is more emphatic in advocating this policy.

Conklin maintains that even in the most distant future there may never appear greater geniuses than Socrates, Plato, Aristotle, Shakespeare, Newton, Darwin, and that "the intellectual evolution of the individual has virtually come to an end, but the intellectual evolution of groups of individuals is only at its beginning." In short, intellectual evolution will become more socialized, the same as industrial evolution (from the productive end), and all other processes to which human beings have seriously applied themselves.

This intellectual evolution will be accomplished, Professor Conklin believes, through increased specialization and cooperation of many individuals. The trend toward specialization is due to the limitation of the brain as a storehouse, which, with knowledge continually increasing and intellectual capacity remaining stationary, permits each individual mind to take in only a small portion of the sum of human knowledge. Therefore, in this age, intellectual specialization is absolutely necessary.

### Heredity and Environment

There is a great deal of speculation regarding the relative influence of heredity and environment. Both are positive forces, the full power of which we can hardly weigh with any degree of accuracy, because of varying circumstances and many unknown or hidden factors involved in each case that may be analyzed.

Darwin held the opinion, as the result of a lifetime of critical observation, that men differ less in capacity than in zeal and determination to utilize the powers they have. Zeal, in a sense, may be considered the successful application of the energetic constitution, the vital nerve force, or the libido of the Freudians. We know that vast quantities of this vital force are squandered or directed along socially non-productive channels, so that even in the case of much intellectual capacity, the results frequently are not satisfactory. The significance of this phase of the question, and the possibilities of prescribing a remedy, will be treated later on.

It is generally agreed that no constant distinction can be recognized between the brain of a philosopher and that of many an unlearned person. Neither size nor weight of brain, nor complexity of convolutions, bears any constant relation to ignorance or intelligence, although it is possible that the specialized microscopist may find differences between the brain of the trained thinker and the untrained individual.

H. H. Goddard (*Psychology of the Normal and Subnormal*, page 63) states: "Even the external appearance of the brain itself shows no condition characteristic of feeble-mindedness. The number of convolutions is not markedly different from the normal. Indeed, of a hundred brains, half of which would be the brains of defectives, ranging from idiocy up, it is probable that no neurologist, however familiar with brain convolutions, would be able to group the brains accurately, not even those of the idiots."

In order to appreciate the complexity of the brain, we might try to grasp that the child at birth has ten billion (10,000,000,000) brain cells or neurons, which number is never increased throughout the life of the individual. The growth and increase is in *size*, not in *number*. And the total growth from birth to physical maturity represents an increase of but four-fold in weight. The brain grows from an average weight of about 360 grams (twelve ounces) at birth to about 1400 grams (three pounds), at the age of twenty. This relatively small increase may better be realized when we compare it with the growth of the entire body, which represents an increase in weight of twenty-three fold—from about six or seven pounds at birth to 140 to 160 pounds at twenty. The new-born baby is, indeed, top-heavy, and the resultant size of his cranium tends to make the process of birth the extreme ordeal it is for the modern mother, particularly of the white race.

A small man with the same size head as a big man will, other things being equal, display more energy. Napoleon's head always appeared to the Dutchesse d'Abrantes to be "too large for his body." Mozart's head was also disproportionately large. Both of these men were physically small, and were noted for the abundance of nerve-energy they displayed. In weight of brain, considerable differences have existed among men of acknowledged power. Whereas the average weight of the male brain is about 48 ounces, Cuvier's weighed 64 ounces; Abercrombie's and Schiller's 64; De Morgan and Gauss, the mathematicians', 52¾ and 52 respectively. But Grote, the historian, had a brain only three-quarters of an ounce above the average, while the brains of Tiedemann, the anatomist, and Hausmann, the mineralogist, fell five and six ounces below it. The heaviest known human brain belonged to a Sussex (England) bricklayer, who died of tuberculosis in University College Hospital in 1849. It exceeded 67 ounces, and was well proportioned. In physique, its owner was not greatly above the average, being five feet nine inches in height and of robust frame. The man could not read or write (which was not unusual for a workingman of his time), though he was said to have had a good memory and was fond of politics.[3]

Havelock Ellis here brings to notice an ingenious psychological consideration when he shows that width of hips is a female characteristic commonly admired by men. Inasmuch as a wide pelvis is one which can accommodate and safely give birth to a large fætal head, this suggests a practical bearing on the eugenics issue.

[3] The following comparisons are of interest in the study of brains: The figures of Thurnam (*On the Weight of the Human Brain*) establish a difference between the brains of Europeans and African negroes of about five ounces. A Bushwoman's brain, examined by Marshall (*Proceedings of the Royal Society*) was found to be remarkably deficient in its convolutions, especially in the occipital, the middle and lower frontal and the temporal regions—a formation which would clearly conduce to poverty of ideas. The human brain of the lowest order, in fact, scales down toward that of the ape. Le Bon estimates the cranial capacity of the gorilla at 600 cubic centimetres, the lowest African or Australian black's at 1200, and the Modern European's at from 1800 to 1900. From this it would appear that some human races are mentally as near to the gorilla as to the highest civilized types.

Large heads mean, in general, large brains and it would be unfortunate for the white race if men admired hips as narrow as those, for instance, of the negress, whose pelvis could not find room for the average head of a pure white baby, and who suffers terribly in many cases where the father is white, especially if the child is a boy.

Although the brains of Cuvier, Gauss and Beethoven were unusually large, they have been matched in size and apparent complexity by the brains of unknown and unlearned persons, one example of which we have just cited. These persons may be said to have been *richly endowed by nature but have never learned to use their talents.* Of course, it is impossible to say whether these individuals, naturally gifted, failed to rise to some approximation of their possibilities be. cause of scant opportunities, insurmountable economic obstacles, or failure to secure a satisfactory adjustment of the vital urge along socially constructive lines.

It has been well said that heredity gives not actualities, but only potentialities. It depends upon circumstances whether they shall become actualities. The circumstances are environment in all its multifarious ramifications.

In *Heredity and Environment,* Conklin states: "A more dreadful though less universal tragedy is the loss of real personalities who have native endowments of genius and leadership but who for lack of proper environmental stimuli have remained undeveloped and unknown; the 'mute, inglorious Miltons' of the world . . . the Newtons, Darwins, Pasteurs who were ready formed by nature but who never discovered themselves. One shudders to think how narrowly Newton escaped being an unknown farmer, or Faraday an obscure bookbinder, or Pasteur a provincial tanner. In the history of the world there must have been many men of equal native endowments who missed the slender chance which came to these.''

This quotation from Professor Conklin is a just recognition of the cultural possibility of man, and of its universality, even if it appears only in spots in its higher form.

It has become an axiom that every great crisis brings forth a great leader—usually one unknown or unrecognized before the circumstances demonstrated his particular fitness and qualifications. This, on the one hand, has been the cause of believing in the old fallacy that great minds appear only at long intervals, because great crises usually appear only at long intervals. On the other hand, it furnishes food for the thought that the intellectual material is always with us, already formed, and requiring only the powerful stimulus of great necessity to develop its potentialities and force universal recognition of the fact.

What a loss to the sum of cultural development and what a retardation of the sciences there was wrought by the blighting suppression of the Middle Ages! A classic instance that has recently received some renewed attention will serve the two-fold purpose of showing how a monumental genius of the thirteenth century was cruelly hampered and his endeavors largely frustrated; and what must have been the effect generally of this policy of blanket suppression of independent thought and research.

Marvellously endowed with intelligence and creative energy, Roger Bacon, the thirteenth century Franciscan friar—born in Somersetshire in 1214—is believed to have anticipated by centuries the principles of a number of sciences. Bacon is considered by the leading medievalists to have been several hundred years ahead of his time in solving some of the problems of modern science. This irrepressible student, having been persecuted, condemned and imprisoned as a necromancer, and forbidden for twenty years to write for publication, was forced to put the more revolutionary results of his research and experimentation into a secret code.[4] The key to these discoveries, inventions and hypotheses was unravelled by Dr. William Romaine Newbold of the

[4] "All great things have been won by men who would not conform. Where would astronomy be now if the great ones had not risked excommunication? Where would the Darwinian theory be if its author had conformed with the views of the majority? Where would. modern surgery stand but for Lister's disregard of the sneers of his opponents? . . . The history of science, and indeed of human thought, proves that men are not grateful to the discoverer of such truths as tend to disturb existing notions. The instinctive tendency of mankind is to resent any disturbance of its placid hold of traditional beliefs, and to muzzle or suppress the disturber."—Bernard Hollander.

University of Pennsylvania, who has succeeded
in transcribing a portion of the old vellum manuscript.

Dr. Newbold, who is averse to making any
sensational statements regarding Bacon's discoveries, informed me that the documents "prove
that he had a telescope and microscope and *saw
many things never seen before and not seen again
for ages.*" It is known that the writings of Bacon
influenced Columbus (over two hundred years
later) in concluding that the earth is round, and
he therefore may be said to have been responsible
for the discovery of America in 1492. Bacon was
the first of the medieval thinkers to grasp the
idea of the *importance of experiment,* and the
main object for which he fought was the emancipation of scientific research from the trammels of
authority.

Here is another example of the unequal contest
between the spirit of the Caveman, as exemplified
in the dominating powers of the thirteenth century, and an isolated individual of rare intellectual capacity. His genius could only function
surreptitiously, restricted as it was by the
strait-jacket conventions of his time. And this
Caveman spirit is still with us today in a degree
scarcely less vindictive—but is directed against
the social, political and industrial non-conformists
of our time—as will be evidenced in subsequent
chapters.

Family histories have been cited to prove the

contention that heredity is a prime factor in producing high intellectual capacity. Perhaps the most interesting case of this kind that has been instanced is the family which produced Charles Darwin, the discoverer of a fundamental principle of biology. His grandfather was Erasmus Darwin, physician, poet and philosopher, and independent expounder of the doctrine of organic evolution. Darwin's father was an eminent physician, described by his son as "the wisest man I ever knew." The maternal grandfather of Darwin was Josiah Wedgwood, the famous founder of the pottery works. His first cousin was Francis Galton, the formulator of the science of eugenics, whose contributions, both direct and by way of stimulating thought among others, are of inestimable benefit to the race. Charles Darwin has five living sons, each a man of distinction, including Francis Darwin and Sir George Darwin, both original thinkers who have high achievements to their credit in the realms of science. It would be difficult to attribute this sequence of brilliancy to pure chance, or to the influence of environment alone, although environmental conditions undoubtedly were factors in the full development of the individuals cited.

As the basis of the cultural side of our personality is essentially the development of our rational qualities, as contrasted with the more or less indiscriminate expression of the emotions, which constitute the primitive side of our nature, we must look for our higher development along the lines of rigorous rational thought. In this connection, Count Alfred Korzybski [5] (*Manhood of Humanity*), a Polish engineer and mathematical philosopher, has formulated a remarkable hypothesis of the rôle of mankind in the realm of nature. If time vindicates the contentions of this painstaking observer and logician, who has applied the exact science and rigid logic of mathematics to the life-expressing forces of nature, he will have rendered a contribution of inestimable value to human knowledge.

It should be emphasized that the fullest development of the cultural possibilities of man does not eliminate the primitive side of his nature—the Caveman within. It rather coordinates into a harmonious working organism forces which generate friction, with all its disastrous results, when they are permitted to work at cross purposes; that is, when they are not understood, or are suffered to be ignored.

The rational method is to develop the higher cultural qualities that are distinctive of man and responsible for his progress, and that have made him the adaptable *master* of his environment (but not yet of himself), and at the same time to give due recognition to the primitive desires in a *socially acceptable way*—to enumerate a few: through athletics and sportsmanlike contests; music, literature and art; diversions that offer an

[5] E. P. Dutton & Co., New York, 1921.

emotional outlet that is not asocial in its results; and, perhaps, most important of all, in a healthy sex life, which can best be achieved through rational sex knowledge and the monogamic relationship. If some such expression is not given to the innate forces that are surging up from the jungle of the past, and that have their roots firmly intrenched within us—that are literally the fundamental part of our being—then they will assert themselves no less, but in abnormal and pathological ways. They will not be denied.

The late Professor Shaler of Harvard University has summarized this lack of coordination in the following words, which are quoted from his book, *The Neighbor:* "It is hardly too much to say that all the important errors of conduct, all the burdens of men or of societies are caused by the inadequacies in the association of the primal animal emotions with those mental powers which have been so rapidly developing (comparatively speaking) in mankind."

### BIBLIOGRAPHY

GALTON, FRANCIS, *Inquiries Into Human Faculty,* New York, 1883.

THOMSON, J. A., *Heredity,* New York.

MORGAN, STURTEVANT, MULLER and BRIDGES, *The Mechanism of Mendelian Heredity,* New York, 1915.

SALEEBY, C. W., *Parenthood and Race Culture,* New York, 1916.

ROBINSON, JAMES H., *An Outline of the History of the Western European Mind,* New York, 1919.

ELLIS, HAVELOCK, *The Problem of Race Regeneration,* New York, 1911.

GODDARD, H. H., *Psychology of the Normal and Subnormal,* New York, 1919.

BATESON, W., *Problems in Genetics,* Yale University Press, 1913.

KELLICOTT, W. E., *The Social Direction of Human Evolution,* New York, 1911.

LOEB, J., *Comparative Physiology of the Brain and Comparative Psychology,* New York, 1900.

RIGNANO, E., *The Inheritance of Acquired Characters,* Chicago, 1911.

KORZYBSKI, ALFRED, *Manhood of Humanity,* New York, 1921.

IRWIN, WILL, *The Next War,* New York, 1921.

CONKLIN, E. G., *Heredity and Environment,* Princeton University Press, 1915.

# CHAPTER IV

## THE CAVEMAN UNMASKED—REVELING IN DREAMS

Tell me for a time your dreams, and I will tell you
what you are within.—E. R. PFAFF.

A NUMBER of typical forms of lapses of the cultural personality, and the ascendency of the primitive, individually and en masse, have been alluded to, and their significance will be treated more thoroughly in other chapters. When the primitive personality asserts itself too pronouncedly in daily life, or reverts too far from the conventional level of civilized standards, and when these transgressions of the individual are of a nature that is socially objectionable, he is considered, according to their degree, irrational, unbalanced, or insane.

Now, everyone at times exhibits tendencies, if only momentarily, that are irrational, or lacking in balance, and sudden attacks of insanity are not rare. And, as I shall later demonstrate, the great majority of people seldom are rational, but rather, through habit, custom and tradition, maintain for the most part a standard of behavior that is recognized as socially acceptable. This standard, although slowly changing, is arbitrary, having evolved through ages of growing human experiences, and is riddled with the shot of trial and error. Nevertheless, it is so rigid that the rationalist who attempts, with any degree of consistency, to bend it in conformity with his ideas, is doomed to earn the derision of the multitude, although in the end some of his suggestions may be adopted.

While the Caveman is constantly bobbing up and down, there are times, even in the most rational and most cultured, when he rises to the ascendency, when he stalks forth unmasked and frequently with powerful effect.

We have reviewed his great past, his vast biological background, and his vital character which demands expression. This expression, in its primitive form, is always ego-centric, and usually socially objectionable. Whatever culture, rationality and social traits we have developed, are bonds that help to subjugate and subordinate him as long as we are conscious and our will power functions.

However, when the bars of consciousness or will are let down, regardless of our culture or rationality, the Caveman asserts himself. This is particularly observable in the instance of intoxication, when the nectar of Bacchus draws aside the restraining influence of the cultural veneer (the mask of civilization, as it were), and the intoxicated person may revert to almost any degree of savagery or even bestiality. In many cases, on account of a less emotional temperament, the regression is simply to an early stage of childhood. The "laughing drunk," and also the "crying drunk," are not uncommon phenomena—or were not before the era of Volstead. Drinking a slight intoxicant—that is, a drink or so of some mild alcoholic beverage, when the individual still retains his decorum—results in a slighter release of the psychic tension, with its well-known exhilarating effect. Even in this case, it is a subtle relief from the rigid requirements of the individual's cultural personality. Often the greater the cultural development, if it involves undue repression, the more pronounced are the reactions when the repression is removed.

Two thousand five hundred years ago, the Greek philosopher Heraclitus said: "For those who are awake, only one universal world exists. During sleep every one returns to his own." We surrender the field of psychic activity to the Caveman when we lapse into sleep. When the tension of consciousness is released, another being (or, more accurately, another side of our personality —the primitive one) comes to the fore. He may act in any way indicative of his great age. He may manifest the characteristics of the man of a few thousands of years back, or of many, many thousands, and perhaps add thereto some of his tendencies of the present. But these tendencies of the present are usually his crass desires. One

thing you can depend upon, he is always fundamentally primitive, irrational, inconsistent, self-
centered, ego-centric, anti-social.[1]

The long systematized repression on the part of
our cultural personality has become an influencing
factor even in our sleep. In that case, the Caveman disguises some of his most objectionable behavior and disports himself in sufficient symbolism to avoid offending the consciousness of his
host, which seems never to be completely relaxed.
On questions that are not connected with a powerful taboo, he will maintain the same supreme indifference to logic, reason and rational discrimination that characterizes him in individuals less
adept in censoring his grosser qualities.

### Age of Dream Interest

People always have been interested in dreams
as far back as human thought is recorded. It is
no exaggeration to say that dreams have profoundly influenced the lives of individuals and the
destinies of nations. Back in the more primitive
days of man, dreams exerted a tremendous influence over his conduct and behavior. The

---

[1] "When we lose consciousness, either in sleep, in delirium, or
under the influence of anaesthetics, our minds are not blank, but
are working rapidly. A person talking in his sleep will give
verbal expression to the most vital wishes, which would shock his
waking mind. They find utterance, but do not enter his own
consciousness. If they do, they are always expressed in symbolic
form."—Elida Evans, *The Problem of the Nervous Child*, Dodd,
Mead & Co., 1920.

elaborate conceptions of mythology, folklore and legendary are now conceded to be the day-dreams of young humanity. They were the dreams of individuals projected upon the nation and in time became a part of the racial culture of their period.

Many of the prominent features and allegories of the great religions of to-day have identically the same characteristics. They, too, were conceived back in the twilight of civilization, when mankind associated his dreams either with divine or diabolic inspiration, and if they appeared to be in the former category, the dreamer was considered appointed as a chosen oracle. All the revealed religions have this common genesis, and their themes are woven around some central character who personifies the power and prerogatives of the mythological Gods.

Innumerable books have been written on the subject, and superstitions, ideas and theories formulated without number concerning dream phenomena. Notwithstanding this vast field that has been so long open for exploration, study and research, it is only within comparatively recent years that any real substantial progress has been made in arriving at a true understanding of the nature of dreams and their manifestations.

The reason for this is the same as may be given for the slow progress in all fields of scientific endeavor. While dreams generally have been associated with the fantastic, the unreal, the supernormal, when, indeed, not with the supernatural, they are now nevertheless connected with a definite branch of science, and consequently, during recent years, great strides have been made in understanding them.

Dream phenomena now have a well established position in the realms of psychology and it is in this field that their study has been placed on a scientific basis. As a matter of fact, a real understanding of psychology requires an understanding of dreams, their language and their significance. This is a wide departure from their former association with the supernatural, as manifestations of the mystic soul element, some detached spirit from within or without, or any one of a hundred other mysterious rôles that were attributed to them. But this again is merely in line with all discoveries of natural forces. An understanding of their nature removes them from the sphere of the supernatural to the natural.

We are constantly impressed with the fact that the ancients, and many people even down to recent times, considered dreams, not a product of the dreamer's own mind, but a divine inspiration —in other words, an extraneous agency working through the individual. The strength of this belief, and its widespread acceptance, could only find a basis because of the fundamental duality of our nature. One side of our nature functions one way during our waking hours, barring the occasional lapses that are less conspicuous, and the other side manifests itself in strange, weird, often unfathomable ways during the period of sleep. This naturally led the dreamer of ancient times, who could not reconcile his dreams with his waking thoughts, to attribute the dreams to a divine, or sometimes diabolic, source.

While Aristotle was the first thinker known to have disputed this contention—and his theories regarding dreams were modifications of the old beliefs rather than purely rational conceptions—the popular belief in the supernatural origin of dreams long survived this Greek sage.

Some of the foremost philosophers, poets and dramatists of modern and near-modern times have shown an excellent working knowledge of dream phenomena, arriving at many of the same conclusions as the scientific observer of today, without apparently employing any definite system or science. Nietzsche, in particular, has given us many salient bits of wisdom concerning the nature of dreams. One of his most profound observations, it seems to me, is summed up in the following words: "In our sleep and in our dreams we pass through the whole thought of earlier humanity. I mean, in the same way that man reasons in his dreams, he reasoned when in the waking state many thousands of years. The first *causa* which occurred to his mind in reference to anything that needed explanation, satisfied him, and passed for truth. In the dream this atavistic relic of humanity manifests its existence within us, for it is the foundation upon which the higher rational faculty developed. The dream carries us back into earlier states of human culture, and affords us a means of understanding them better"—(*Human, All too Human*).

Shakespeare frequently used reference to dreams to make telling points, or to illustrate the psychic bent in his characters. The following bit of dialogue, only one of several instances from *Hamlet* alone, offers an interesting study of two contrasting types:

> *Hamlet:*—O God, I could be bounded in a nutshell and count myself a king of infinite space, were it not that I have bad dreams.

> *Guildenstern:*—Which dreams indeed are ambition; for the very substance of the ambitious is merely the shadow of a dream.

In *Hamlet,* the genius of Shakespeare has given us an illuminating study of a neurotic type, with an outstanding, unconscious mother-fixation, or Œdipus complex, which he consciously tried to compensate for by denouncing his mother for her folly. The psychic conflict which this involved must assuredly have produced distressing dreams.

The practical Guildenstern recognized the self-centered, egotistic nature of the dream, which in normal life, as well as the abnormal, is bound up irretrievably with the ambitions. The dream expresses more than any other psychic operation the potency of the desires—and desires are ambitions. The actual nature of the desires or wishes may not always be understood, particularly in adult life, when the individual labours under so many repressions and inhibitions, with the accompanying highly charged organism of powerful urges and primitive emotions. The child, however, being less repressed by the inhibitions of its environment, and not yet experiencing the more compelling force of those urges which rapidly develop from puberty, dreams of its simpler wishes in an undisguised form.

## Plain Wish Fulfilment

The dreams of young children have been found to be primarily related to food, good things to eat and drink, and particularly when withheld from them. Coveted toys are also a common theme of childhood dreams. The child's dreams are very vivid, and so realistic that it often thinks that its desires actually have been realized. Disappointment and denial act as a stimulation to dreams; the reality of the latter in general being closely related to the extent of the former.

Freud cites a characteristic example to illustrate this point. His little nephew, only twenty-two months old, was given the honour of handing him a small basket of cherries on his birthday. It proved to be a difficult task for the little fellow to let the basket go, and he kept repeating, "Cherries in it!" But his compensation was as real to him as his disappointment was keen. He had, for some time previously been in the habit of telling his mother each morning that he had dreamt of the "white soldier," an officer in a white cloak whom he had once looked upon with admiration on the street. On the day after the birthday incident, he joyfully announced upon awakening that "Herman ate up all the cherries!" which idea could only have originated in a dream.

The strength of impression of children's dreams is shown by a test of Dr. C. W. Kimmins of London, who discovered through a period of dream-study covering several years and involving six thousand children, that boys and girls between eight and sixteen have the power of graphic description of their dreams that "so far exceeds their ability in ordinary essay writing on topics selected by the teacher that it would appear as if some fresh mental element had come into play." The explanation is simple. They dream of things that interest them. The teacher's subjects are not always so interesting.

Even in adult life, where the denial suffered is very great, and the desires are pressing and continuous, the dreams may be vividly presented in the manner of infantile wish-fulfilment. Perhaps no better illustration of this can be cited than that instanced by Otto Nordenskjold in his book, *Antarctic* (1904). He states that the vivid dreams of the crew were very characteristic of their inmost thoughts. Even those with whom dreams

had formerly been an exception had long stories
to tell when dream experiences were exchanged
in the morning. Eating and drinking formed the
central point around which most of the dreams
were grouped. (They were living on a very restricted diet of canned and salted foods.) There
were dreams of whole mountains of tobacco; of
ships approaching on the open sea under full sail;
of a letter carrier bringing mail and giving a long
explanation of why he had been so long delayed,
that he had delivered the mail at the wrong place,
and only after great effort had he been able to
get it back. In this time of great privation, which
was unconsciously compensated for by wish-fulfilment in dreams, Nordenskjold comments as follows on the psychological factor in the case:
"But one can readily understand how we longed
for sleep. It alone could afford us everything
that we most ardently desired."

The wish-fulfilment character of dreams has
been widely noted outside of Freudian psychology.
There is the old Chinese proverb: "The prisoner
dreams of freedom; the thirsty of springs of
water." A Hungarian proverb recognizes the
universality of the same propensity by applying
it to the animal world: "The pig dreams of
acorns; the goose of maize."

So-called prophetic and inspirational dreams
have led, seemingly, to very far-reaching results,
and are the cause of endless discussion. They
have been undoubtedly the cause of many, if not

all, religious cults and sects and numerous theories that have been set forth for the approbation of man. On account of our comparatively limited knowledge of the unconscious mind, from which dreams emanate, it is difficult to ascertain all the facts and therefore unwise to draw dogmatic conclusions.

In approaching this phase of the subject from the scientific angle, we must recognize that many factors are involved, some of which we have yet to become acquainted with. It is well to bear in mind, however, that countless incidents which have been a part of our experience are soon lost to memory, and many more are not consciously observed at all. This vast accumulation of sensory experiences, which is ever being added to, does not form a static part of our psychic content. It is constantly working itself around, popping out here and there, usually in unrecognized forms, in curious blendings and grotesque effects, as we so often experience in our dreams.

### So-Called Prophetic Dreams

After every tragic accident or disaster, people rush forward and give utterance to a prophetic dream they had purporting to foretell the occurrence. These people are undoubtedly honest in their belief, though rarely analytic in reviewing the circumstances. A great ocean steamship sinks, and we have the testimony of those who had visualized the catastrophe in a dream. How do the circumstances fit in with the facts? We recognize that we have all sorts of fantastic, incoherent dreams, usually involving many seemingly unrelated factors. Out of millions of people, probably some—even many—will dream of ships in any given night. The tragedy occurs, and instantly those who had dreamt of a ship of any kind will recall the incident; then the deeper they go into the details of their dream as the day wears on and after they have read of the particulars concerning the loss of the ship, the more they will note the points of similarity.

In the first place, the mere fact that they had dreamt of a ship, with which was probably associated a mass of hazy dream material that by a slight stretch of the imagination could be conjured into corroborating details, leads them to believe that their dream has been prophetic. In the second place, the variety of news they have absorbed on the subject immediately afte, e accident becomes known, is confused with the dream memories and easily supplements them, thus doubly proving to the dreamer that he had been appraised of the coming event through a supernatural source.

Even more convincing testimony than this is usually cited in the event of such a disaster. There are always people who come forward, invariably relatives or close friends of those who have perished, who can prove that they warned the victims not to sail, as they had forebodings of impending danger which originated in a dream. They have uttered their fears publicly in the presence of witnesses before the ship sailed.

What are the circumstances that must be taken into consideration in cases like this, before one can feel justified in drawing a fair conclusion? It is likely that a ship has never left port with her human cargo without some nervous individuals—relatives or friends near and dear to those embarking—having expressed their fears for the safety of the trip. In nine thousand nine hundred and ninety-nine cases out of ten thousand, nothing happens to confirm these predictions, and we hear no more of them. The nervous individuals proceed to find an outlet for their anxiety in more responsive channels. In the one case in ten thousand or more, when an accident, trivial or disastrous, occurs, we have the inevitable testimony of those who had foreseen the danger in a dream and forewarned the unfortunates. As Lord Bacon observed: "Men mark when they hit, but not when they miss."

This line of thought could be carried on without end, and is applicable to innumerable other misfortunes, such as train wrecks, fires, drownings through bathing or boating, automobile accidents, and so on. What mother is there who does not think many times a day of the danger of her child on the street from vehicular traffic, and who is not constantly warning the young one to look out for the automobiles. When an accident does occur, as so many accidents of this kind do every day throughout the country, the mother's mind instantly recurs to a certain feeling of mistrust she had at a certain time, and in her distracted state of mind, a commonplace psychological incident that she has doubtless experienced every day for years is distorted into a premonition.

All these factors relating to dreams, with their endless complications and associations with past experiences, mostly long forgotten, are a part of the constant stream of undirected thought that is passing through the mind of each individual all the time, asleep or awake. These psychic manifestations are extensive enough, and rich enough in highly coloured material, to furnish a ready-made premonition or forewarning to fit the circumstances of any accident or misfortune that may happen. Fortunately, in comparison with the fears, they rarely happen, and we seldom feel called upon to announce our pre-enlightenment; but when the occurrence takes place, the premonitory and prognostic omen is never wanting.

The very nature of the phenomena I have outlined implies a duality of personality, which has been variously designated as the *conscious* and the *unconscious*, the *rational* and the *mystic*, the *objective* and the *subjective*, the *mortal* and the *spiritual*. When fully analysed, however, all this simmers down to a highly ramified organism that binds the very remote past with the present. This fusion of the archaic and the modern, when not reasonably complete and coordinated, results in internal conflict and disintegration. Many forms of hysteria, some with their mystic demonstrations, are merely examples of dissociation of personality.

At the same time, I am not the dogmatist to assert that there never have been cases of genuine premonition, or that mental telepathic communication is impossible. I would say, rather, that the great mass of evidence that is alleged to prove these contentions is farfetched, when not spurious on its face. I have never myself experienced, nor observed in others with whom I have been in personal touch, any "premonitions" that were not obviously a link in a chain of associations. And I have made diligent, painstaking efforts to get into telepathic communication with different individuals, but always with absolutely negative results.

There is a not uncommon type of dream wherein we seem suddenly to solve a difficult problem that has long puzzled our mind and defied all our intellectual resources. Bookkeepers who have searched their accounts in vain for an error have seen the mistake in a dream, and have thus been able to turn to the exact page of their books and find the elusive troublemaker. Professor Hilprecht had spent much time trying to decipher two small fragments of agate, supposedly finger rings, from the temple of Bel in ancient Babylonia. He had given up the task and classified the pieces as undecipherable in the manuscript of a book on the subject. One night he approved the final proofs of his book with a feeling of dissatisfaction on account of his inability to solve the cipher on the ancient stones. He retired to bed and had a vivid dream: A priest of Nippur appeared and led him to the treasure chamber of the temple of Bel and told him that the two fragments should be put together, as they were not finger rings, but earrings made for a god by cutting a cylinder into three parts. The next morning he went to his agate fragments, put them together as suggested in the dream, and read the inscription with little difficulty.

There are two important considerations involved in dreams of this general nature. The first is that our mind really takes in all the circumstances connected with our experiences, but only a small portion of them is subject to our rational discrimination. In the instance of the bookkeeper, it can only be assumed that in poring over his book, in a preoccupied manner, he had *unconsciously* noted the error, and it was only when the tension of consciousness was released, when the unconscious mind had free play, that the mistake was revealed to him. It had been impressed on the negative of the unconscious mind, and when conditions were favorable, this impression was projected back to the foreconscious in such a way as to be visualized in the dream. The same general situation holds in the difficulty of Professor Hilprecht.

The second factor that contributes to the solution of problems in dreams is that in our sleep the excessive concentration of attention is released, which enables the mind to sift through a vast number of possibilities. Concentration is a necessary force in any line of activity, but there are special instances when it does not give the best results. It tends to narrow the mental horizon and limits the scope of reasoning to one specific channel. Inside of the specific channel on which the mind is concentrated, the faculties are intensified with results that are normally in proportion. Furthermore, when we concentrate on a task we are apt to be convinced that the solution lies in a certain mode of action, and we bar out suggestions that would tend to throw some added light on the subject.

We often unconsciously realize the necessity of breaking the tension of concentration when we reach a point that baffles us in working on a problem. Concentration has narrowed our view, and we seek to relax it. We assume an abstract attitude of mind, think of nothing in particular for a few minutes (which means that we permit our unconscious mind to run along at will in its own free channels) in the hope that with relaxation some ideas will pop into consciousness. Jastrow has remarked that when people try hard to recall something, they are apt to scratch the head, rub the chin, tap the table, etc., which tend to produce abstraction, so favorable for letting in new ideas.

### Indicating Physical Ailments

There are dreams, too, that have a decided value in warning us of approaching physical indispositions and unhealthy conditions. Some of these, with less knowledge of our physiological functions, would be extremely difficult to analyse and might seem mystical indeed.

H. Addington Bruce, in *Sleep and Sleeplessness,* has described one of his own dreams which illustrates this point. He says that at least twenty times during a period of six months he had the same dream—namely, that a cat was clawing at his throat. There might be some variation in the setting, but the central episode was always the same, and usually the fury of the cat's attack was so great that it would awaken him. He was very much puzzled over the recurring dream, and attributed it to indigestion, finally accepting it as an ordinary nightmare.

One day as a result of a heavy cold that settled in his throat, he submitted to a medical examination which, to his great surprise, revealed the presence of a growth requiring immediate surgical treatment. Sometime later it occurred to him that after the removal of the dangerous growth, he had not again been troubled by the cat-clawing dream. He had suffered no pain, nor the least inconvenience from the growth in his throat, and was not in the slightest measure conscious of its presence.

Galen (*Prophecy in Dreams*) mentions the case of a man who dreamed that his leg was turned to stone, and a few days later developed a paralysis of the leg.

Aristides, the Greek orator, is said to have dreamed in the temple of Æsculapius, where the old Greeks were accustomed to go for inspirational dreams, that a bull attacked and wounded him in the knee. On awakening he found evidence of a tumor growing there.

Conrad Gessner dreamed that he was stung by a serpent. A few days later a so-called plague-boil developed on his breast as a result of which he died.

Hammond cited the case of a patient who, for two nights before an attack of hemiplegia, dreamed that he was cut in two from chin to perineum. Soon after he was afflicted with paralysis.

All dreams of this type are due to some reaction of the autonomic nervous system to the slight irritating stimulus, not consciously perceived, of the pathological condition. A more common illustration of this is the dream of dental trouble or tooth extraction, so often found to have its origin in a blind pus pocket, which an X-ray picture will confirm. Dental dreams also are believed to be induced by erotic stimuli.

### Typical Dreams

Among the types of commonplace dreams are those of falling and of flying. There are various causes attributed to these dreams. And as they are so universal, it seems reasonable that there must be certain definite biological and psychological factors that instigate them.

Flying dreams are doubtless due primarily to man's long desire to soar through the air like the birds, whose faculty in this particular he has always envied. This is a simple wish-fulfilment, and we have noted how potent desires are in influencing the unconscious mind. Another causative factor attributed to flying dreams is the rhythmic rising and falling of the chest when one sleeps in a certain position. Still another, is the symbolical version, which indicates that the dreamer aspires to greater heights of achievement and to rise above his fellows. It is a manifestation of the ego urge, so powerful in us all.

Falling dreams are frequently very terrifying, and are usually associated with the nightmare group. Some biologists have offered the theory that the falling dream is a racial memory, an heritage of the ape-man who lived in the trees. In these dreams we always catch ourselves, land safely or wake up in the excitement, which indicates that our progenitor, who originally experienced the shock which caused this indelible psychic impression that has become a biological fixture, also caught himself or fell to comparative safety, else the impression could not have been carried down.

The symbolical explanation is also given: That the dreamer, whose censorship over his fore-conscious is on the alert even in his sleep, dreams of falling as a disguised form of satisfying an ethically forbidden wish, sexual or otherwise. The dream represents a "fall from grace," and satisfies an unconscious desire to revert to a primitive state, and to be temporarily relieved from the oppressive restrictions of modern society.[2]

It is probable that most falling dreams are childhood memories lived over in our sleep. Every child has fallen little or much. It is one of the hardships the infant must undergo in learning to walk. It is obvious that some of these falls are a powerful shock to the nervous system—which appears never to forget an experience—thus leaving a permanent impression. Even many years after, some stimulus may arouse in the psychic stream a recollection of the fall, which is registered in the form of a dream.

Dreams which are concerned with entering into, or emerging from, water or hurriedly passing through narrow spaces, usually associated with fear, are believed to be based upon biochemical

---

[2] "The sliding down is likely to symbolize the sexual act; the waters are probably the amniotic liquor which appear so frequently in the dreams of women."—Walter Samuel Swisher, *Religion and the New Psychology.*

memories of the embryonic life, the prenatal period in the mother's womb, and the act of birth. The water in which the dreamer imagines himself is invariably perfectly suited to his temperature, representing the amniotic or uterine fluid. The journey is through a dark and narrow passage-way, symbolizing the uterus and vagina; and the sensation of being forced from the rear corresponds to the act of birth, finally emerging into the open. The fear, too, is analogous to the reaction of the new-born infant who, coming from its abode of perfect serenity and comfort, and plunged into a world of new and foreboding sensations, for the first time experiences fear.

A universal similarity has been observed in the content of dreams of this type, which leads to the conclusion that they are derived from the unconscious memories of the organism in the universal experience of embryonic life and birth. Again the analogy of dreams and mythology intrudes itself upon us. The birth of many mythological characters, such as Adonis, Osiris and Bacchus is associated with a watery setting, and there is the well-known legend of Moses' origin in the chronicles of the Hebrews.

Dreams of death to a parent or other loved one are very common; as also are nakedness, or so-called embarrassment dreams. This latter type is considered an exhibitionist quality revived in the Unconscious. Exhibitionism is an attribute of infancy, as it was of the infancy of the race, and the ancients paid attention enough to it to immortalize the theme. The mythological conception of Narcissus, who fell in love with the reflection of himself in a pool, is still kept alive in art and literature, and the present-day popular use of the mirror indicates that this trait has not died out.

No summary of dreams would be complete without alluding to the common anxiety-dream or nightmare. This form of dream picture, accompanied by anxiety, represents the subject (usually female) pursued by a dangerous beast which threatens to throw itself on the dreamer. Characteristically, it is frequently a stallion or bull—animals which long have stood as symbols of the potent strength of animal masculinity. The Freudians see in these animal figures the symbolized givers of sexual satisfaction, denied in conscious thinking. Another symbolization aiming at this end appears in dreams of burglars who, armed with revolvers, daggers or similar weapons, press in upon the dreamer. Dr. E. Hitschmann remarks: "The starting up from sleep because of such anxiety-dreams, one finds frequently in widows and ungratified women as a characteristic kind of disturbance in sleep."

The full significance of this interpretation of anxiety-dreams is only appreciated when one has made a study of symbolism and its relation to sexual phenomena. Dr. Ernest Jones maintains that "there are probably more symbols of the male genital organ than all other symbols put together." The person who dreams of a snake, a dagger, a fish or a bird, does not regard these objects as a phallic symbol and is usually unwilling to accept this conclusion until the logic of dream analysis convinces him. This is realized more fully when we refer to the history of phallic symbolism.

Countless variations of these themes occur in the mythology, folklore and legends of all periods, and they are an ever recurring feature in the motifs of literature and the arts. We find the snake alone a phallic symbol in unnumbered instances. Sometimes it creeps into the mouth, or it bites the breast like Cleopatra's legendary asp. In the notable pictures by Franz Stuck, snakes bear the significant titles, "Vice," "Sin," "Lust." One of a number of excellent poetic examples embodying this motif is given in Mörike's charming lyric: [3]

*The Maiden's First Love Song*
What's in the net?
Behold,
But I am not afraid;
Do I grasp a sweet eel,
Do I seize a snake?
Love is a blind
Fisherwoman;
Tell the child
Where to seize—
Already it leaps in my hands.

[3] Quoted from *Psychology of the Unconscious,* by C. G. Jung, Moffat, Yard & Co., Pub.

Ah, Pity, or delight!
With nestlings and turnings
  It coils on my breast,
  It bites me, oh, wonder!
  Boldly through the skin,
  It darts under my heart.
Oh, Love, I shudder!

  What can I do, what can I begin?
    That shuddering thing;
    There it crackles within
    And coils in a ring.

    It must be poisoned.
    Here it crawls around.
  Blissfully I feel as it worms
    Itself into my soul
    And kills me finally.

Nothing in normal life reveals our dual nature better than dreams. That there is a crude, irrational, archaic side to us is amply proved by them. And there are some outstanding themes in dreams, common to all the people and races of the earth, regardless of language, customs, social development, or time. Since the ancient days when dreams were first observed and recorded, they have caused mankind no end of wonderment.

### Sleep—Normal Regression of Primitive Self

There is very good reason to believe that sleep is necessary as a means of temporarily relaxing the psychic tension; that is, enabling us to revert regularly to that stage which in the race is represented in prehistoric ages; and in the individual, in his prenatal state—rather than to secure "rest" and to "repair the wear and tear" of the organism.

Space will permit only a brief and inadequate analysis of this hypothesis, but a few suggestive thoughts will lend confirmation to it. From all known physiological considerations, fatigue should be as well relieved by assuming a restful position for the body and suspending all physical and mental effort, as in sleep.

If sleep was required primarily for rest and the repair of tissue, then the duration of sleep on an average would be conditioned by the expenditure of energy. The truth is that those who expend the most energy usually sleep less than those who expend little. And energetic persons sleep *less* when they are active than when they are not utilizing their energy to capacity.

This is explained by the fact that those persons who are of a more primitive nature, must revert more frequently or for longer periods to the primitive life which is assured in sleep. It is not essentially a case of fatigue and recuperation, but the primitive psychological state demands more frequent ·access to a primitive psychological environment—which is afforded only in sleep. The Caveman insists upon returning regularly to his native Caveland, which he can only do when the bars of consciousness are removed.

The various parts of the organism are performing their functions quite as diligently in sleep as when one is awake and occupying the same position. On the other hand, extreme fatigue is not conducive to sleep. We have all been at times "too tired to sleep." And, as I have stated, people who lead inactive, indolent or primitive lives, and expend little energy, sleep longer than those who are actively engaged in some effective work.

Examples are often cited of very active men, who expend enormous energy, and sleep very little. Napoleon, during the most active years of his career as the conqueror of a great part of Europe, slept only four or five hours out of the twenty-four. When he was banished to St. Helena, living a most inactive life, he slept over twice as long. The short period of sleep of Thomas Edison, a man of vast energy, is likewise well known. A great many other active people, not so prominent in the public notice, also sleep much less than the accepted normal period of eight hours, while less advanced types of individuals, and children, who represent a more primitive stage of development, sleep considerably more than eight hours.

Sleep, according to this hypothesis, is a normal, socially acceptable, means of escaping from reality and gratifying the primitive desires of the Unconscious. The neurotic attempts to flee from reality through his neurosis, as well as through

sleep. On account of the character of our biological make-up, and the insatiable demands of
the primitive side of our nature, we must with
some degree of regularity dissociate ourselves
from our highly artificial environment. The
normal way to accomplish this is in dreams—for
sleep enables the unconscious mind to indulge its
primitive desires by reveling in dreams. And we
all dream continuously throughout our sleep, although we do not ordinarily remember what we
have dreamed.

It is in this way that the strain of the demands
which society makes upon us is alleviated for the
time being. We are psychologically active, in a
primitive way, in our sleep, and we sleep in order
to dream, for dreams relieve the pressure that
accumulates in the act of battling with reality.

### Day Dreams

Day dreams, or phantasying, like their near-
relations of our sleep, are also wish fulfilments.
They indicate what we are striving for, and represent a tendency on the part of the primitive
side of our personality to retreat from the stern
demands of our environment while still maintaining consciousness. We sleep only eight hours,
more or less, out of the twenty-four. The Caveman within us cannot wait for this coveted period
to come around, so he catches us off guard, and
steals a little time between.

In day dreams we realize and enjoy for a few brief moments the unattainable. We have all "built castles in the air." Some of us have soared to untold heights, if only to come down with a crash, when we find reality staring us in the face again. Wishing is one of the most universal of human experiences. We cannot wait for sleep to indulge promiscuously in wishes, so we engage in little wish sprees while seemingly awake. We may not actually be awake to anything but our phantasies. Wishes are as common to the beggar as to the prince or millionaire—perhaps more so, for the former has more to wish for that would enhance his condition of life.

It is true that, unlike the dreams of our sleep, day dreams are usually accompanied by some conscious effort. We tend to guide them, although this tendency in many instances is more apparent than real, as there is also the influence of the unconscious mind—the primitive self—leading us on, whereas we may believe we are directing it.

There are both good and bad features about day dreams. If we develop the power to co-operate with the unconscious psychic forces and "exploit" them through carrying out in reality the more constructive ideas they suggest to us, we are on the way to accomplishing something worth while in life. The evil side of day dreaming is in indulging in it purely as an end in itself, as a primitive psychological pleasure. This gets us nowhere.

To quote from another work of mine, "As a result of reveries or day dreams, combined with some directed thinking, the poet and the artist create their immortal works; the inventor gives to the world his epoch-making mechanical devices; the scientist discovers the natural laws of the universe and utilizes the knowledge so gained for human progress; the ambitious student is inspired and spurred on to reach some goal of constructive effort. Such dreams have resulted in imperishable works of art and literature, great scientific and mechanical achievements, and other priceless accomplishments."

The negative side of day dreaming is in letting the dreams run away with us. This they naturally tend to do, if we give way to our primitive self. The alternative is to direct the dream-stream to an ideal objective, and conquer it for a purpose.

The victims of day dreaming are represented by the loafer of all types and degrees. All lazy, indolent people work incessantly at this unproductive occupation. They do not *act* to realize their ambitions, their dreams. The dreams are both the aspirations and the fulfilment. They simply live their wishes in their dreams, instead of trying to *shape* them in reality.

Children, until taught by example and precept, or forced by circumstances, are much given to day dreaming when not engaged in play or performing simple duties suitable to their age and capabilities. Even the latter soon become irksome, and

they are shunted for play, which is also an expression of the primitive nature. So we see how
the child is dominated almost completely by its
elementary urges. In most cases, it is merely
a question of environmental conditions whether
he will dream himself down into a loafer or up
into communion with the gods and become a
creator of something worth while.

In a word, day dreaming in moderation is desirable under certain conditions. Its abuse is the
abomination.

The chronic victim of this habit finds his
pleasure in dreaming, and he usually prefers to
be alone so that his dreams may not be disturbed.
Thus, he becomes egocentric, anti-social. He flees
from the demands of reality whenever the
occasion presents itself, and he is always anxious
to make such occasions. He seeks refuge from
unbearable actualities in the unreal world of his
dreams. As a result, no matter how shiftless or
lazy; no matter how low he has fallen in the social
scale, his dreams enable him to realize, while they
last, a coveted goal of superiority.

The fairy tales of his childhood come true again
in his dreams—for fairy tales have a literal value
to the child-mind. The most absurd desires are
momentarily realized, and the dreamer is invariably the favored fairy prince, the lavish-living
millionaire, the prodigal son of a bountiful fate.
He has regressed to the infantile level of his
primitive personality, which can find satisfaction

only in the unreal world of dreams. And as it is with boys, so with girls; how many of them have not had their Cinderella dreams?

## BIBLIOGRAPHY

ABRAHAM, KARL, *Dreams and Myths*, Nervous and Mental Disease Monograph Series No. 28.

BRUCE, H. ADDINGTON, *Sleep and Sleeplessness*, Boston.

CORIAT, I., *The Meaning of Dreams*, Boston, 1915.

FREUD, SIGMUND, *The Interpretation of Dreams*, New York, 1914.

MAEDER, A. E., *The Dream Problem*, Nervous and Mental Disease Monograph Series No. 22.

HALL, B., *The Psychology of Sleep*, New York.

MAURY, A., *Le Sommeil et les Rêves*, Paris, 1878.

FIELDING, WILLIAM J., *Psycho-Analysis—The Key to Human Behavior.* Chapter II, Girard, Kansas, 1921.

TRIDON, ANDRÉ, *Psycho-Analysis, Sleep and Dreams*, New York, 1921.

WALSH, WILLIAM S., *The Psychology of Dreams*, New York, 1920.

MANACÉINE, M. DE, *Sleep, its Physiology, Pathology, Hygiene and Psychology*, New York.

CONSTABLE, FRANK C., *Myself and Dreams*, New York, 1920.

ELLIS, HAVELOCK, *The World of Dreams*, London, 1911.

FREUD, SIGMUND, *Delusion and Dream*, New York, 1917.

RANK, OTTO, *The Myth and the Birth of the Hero*, Nervous and Mental Disease Monograph Series No. 18.

# CHAPTER V

## THE CAVEMAN'S DIVERSIONS

But the Old Adam is conservative; he repeats himself mechanically in every child who cries and loves sweets and is imitative and jealous. Reason, with its tragic discoveries and restraints, is a far more precarious and personal possession than the trite animal experience and the ancestral grimaces on which it supervenes; and automatically even the philosopher continues to cut up his old capers, as if no such thing as reason existed.—GEORGE SANTAYANA, *The Comic Mask.*

BESIDES his regular indulgence in revelries, which normally the Caveman finds in dreams (and abnormally in neuroses, insanity and other pathological mental states), he insists upon having his frequent rounds of diversions. These practices, like all other manifestations of our primitive personality, are a means of relaxing the psychic tension, of relieving ourselves from the strain of directed thought and, to a large extent, withdrawing ourselves from the cultural grooves of reason and logic.

There is, however, one fundamental difference between the antics of the Caveman in all other of his manifestations and those which I will sum up as his diversions. While all the former come under the head of egotistical, self-centered and often positively anti-social expressions, the diversions usually are of a social character, involving relations with other persons, and often contributing much to the common weal.

In dreams, whether of the sleep or day variety, the dreamer alone experiences them. They enable him to withdraw into an individual world of his own, and in them he is the chief and central character, to whom all other persons and things are subordinated.

The diversions, on the other hand, not only permit social intercourse, but they require the corroboration of other individuals to achieve their end. Among the most important forms of diversions, or means of gratifying the more social side of our primitive personality, are amusement, sports, play, travel, adventure, humor, jokes, and all other similar classifications.

Every one of these means of expression, and others of their general nature, is a form of obtaining relief from the demands of our highly organized environment. And by occasionally obtaining this relief from our grind in the treadmill of the social organization, we are better able to meet the demands made upon us and maintain our efficiency. Those who very rarely obtain this relaxation from concentrated effort voluntarily are apt to obtain it later in a pathological form, when the Caveman may break loose in obsessions, psychoneuroses, or even fits of insanity.

The safety valve for blowing off the accumulation of psychic steam must be kept in working order, or an explosion is bound to occur sooner or later.

Children, who have not yet developed far along the paths of rationality, spend the greater part of their waking hours in play or other diversions, because their primitive organism requires an almost continuous outlet of the primitive emotions. The child displaying a marvelously energetic capacity for play may become weary, listless and depressed by even the most moderate demand of concentrated attention or application of thought. The prime coat of its civilized veneer is yet in the process of being applied, and until it is on and sticks, the child is the unmasked savage survival. It is in all respects the literal Caveman in a transformed, modern environment, which accounts for so many of the open conflicts between the child and its surroundings.

The difference between the conflicts of the child and those of the average adult is largely one of intensity, as with the development of the individual there is a loss of plasticity. The conflicts are forever recurring, but in adulthood they are more disguised than are those which trouble the child. There is also the inevitable attempt to rationalize them by seeking an excuse for our own shortcomings, mistakes and lack of adaptation, in the acts and omissions of others.

### Wit and Humor

The most common of all the Caveman's diversions are humor and wit—real or attempted—because they are the most accessible. The smallest group of persons, even down to a bare couple, makes it possible to indulge in a witticism, tell a joke, or relate a humorous story. However, a listener is a necessary party to a joke. Shakespeare realized this when he said, in *Love's Labour's Lost* (Act V, Scene 2):

> A jest's prosperity lies in the ear
> Of him that hears it, never in the tongue
> Of him that makes it.

The social value of these expressions of our more elementary nature, which contribute to the well-being of the group, lies in making life more pleasant and agreeable—oftentimes when it is depressing, and again when it would be quite unbearable.

Humor is frequently invoked under very trying or even tragic circumstances. We have all heard of instances when a grim joke has been sprung by some one in a perilous position. It invariably relieves the tension in a crisis or at a serious climax. Notwithstanding a realization of the desperateness, or even hopelessness, of the situation, the relief we experience in a joke under these circumstances often lifts us out of an agonizing suspense. If only temporary, the relief is nevertheless real, and may be a valuable psychic bracer to sustain us in a time of need.

In the presence of death or of some inescapable fate impending, this tendency is quite universal. There is the story of the rogue who, on being led to the gallows on Monday, remarked: "Yes, this week is beginning well."

Soldiers before battle, and in the thick of the fight, are known to relieve the suspense by some expression of wit, however grim. It is an established fact in psychiatry that soldiers who are capable of so relaxing their pent-up emotions or psychic tension are less susceptible to shell-shock.

Indeed, shell-shock, is a form of psychosis produced by an abnormal environment, in which the victim is unable to obtain relief from the intense strain over a prolonged period. Consequently, he develops shell-shock, which is a psychosis or form of insanity that may be of almost any degree of severity, as a substitute form of gratification of the self-preservation urge. It is one of nature's marvelous ways of obtaining compensation in a crisis. It is none the less remarkable on account of its abnormality. It has to be abnormal, because it has been produced by a combination of abnormal circumstances.

Furthermore, it is always successful, from nature's standpoint. The attack makes the victim useless for military service, and sometimes for any other kind, so he is sent to a hospital or other institution. Even if not at once removed, he no longer suffers from the agonizing suspense of bombardment. By a very abnormal process, he has been relieved.

The Irish wake is an old custom that offers an example of relieving the tension in the midst of death. This ancient folk tradition of the Irish race makes full allowances for the psychic needs of the occasion by permitting light story-telling and other expressions of a diverting nature. These practices unconsciously recognize a basic requirement of the psychic make-up.

Wit, humor and the like are forms of mental recreation because they are in substance illogical. And as logic is a development of the conscious mind, or the cultural personality, the interruption of concentration, the deviation from logical reasoning and serious application, affords momentary relaxation.

The characteristic of wit is its brevity, its quick action, its spontaneity. "A flash of wit" in its true sense is as well phrased as "a flash of lightning." Attempted wit, that results in long, studied dissertations, no matter how carefully prepared, is rarely, if ever, wit. While it may sometimes involve humorous situations, there is seldom present the outstanding characteristic of wit.

There is often a deep unconscious significance behind slang phrases and sayings that have grown into the vernacular and colloquial usage. Our primitive nature is still vindictive toward those

who displease or offend us, and such remarks as
"Devil take you," while consciously uttered as a
jest, have to the Caveman a grim connotation.
The following words of a well-known soldier song
did not become popular without a very good
reason:

> Some day I'm going to murder the bugler,
> Some day they are going to find him dead.

In singing this there is a form of compensation
gained by the soldier who so often has been awakened from sleep by the disturbing notes of the
reveille. The unconscious death-wish that is prevalent in other forms of humor, or ill-humor, slang
and oaths, has an interesting psychological background.

### Primitive Wit

The conceptions of wit are as varied as the types
of mentality that engage in it. Among the more
primitive races, groups and individuals, whose
faculties of logic are only crudely developed, wit
has a meaning quite different from that of the
higher types of humanity. What would be a joke
to one type, would have a totally different significance to another.

To illustrate the point in everyday life, we note
the "funny" remarks that infants three or four
years of age are prone to make. They amuse us
because of the generally illogical character of their
statements. In the case of unintentional misuse of

words, resulting in a ludicrous effect, the child
sees nothing humorous, because the infantile mind
lacks the perception to realize that the utterance
is illogical.

However, the child has an appreciation of fun
and humor—which cannot rise above the level of
its primitive personality. The child or person of
comparatively undeveloped mind laughs at what
he believes to be a joke when he is placed in a position of apparent superiority. When the father
gets down on the floor on all-fours, and his infant
youngster grabs his coat-tails or rides on his back,
and bids him assume the lowly function of the
quadruped, the child is conscious of a feeling of
superiority—as the adult is when driving a horse.
This substitute form of superiority, which is
gained when another is subordinated, is quite real
to the primitive mind, and is intensely gratifying
to it.

The characteristic of this psychology is noted
when inferior adult persons laugh or experience
satisfaction at the fall or mishap of someone else.
The you-are-down-and-I-am-up thought (oftentimes only unconsciously realized) is an important
psychologcal factor in all phases of life. A substantial part of the human race receives no incon-
siderable share of its substitute gratification in
some variation of this theme. It is the basic motive of all the witch-hunting, lynching, torturing,
hounding and persecution of the past ages and
the present.

The ignorant fanatic of the Middle Ages, who piled the faggots around the blistering flesh of a Bruno, felt himself lifted to a plane of real importance. The renowned Bruno, who had dared to explore channels of uncharted thought, was at *his* mercy. Think of the possibilities of this satisfaction to the primitive mind! And today we have our Brunos who commit the heresies of holding unpopular opinions and advocating unpopular ideas. These people, too, are meeting the fate of persecution, differing only in degree from that meted out to their prototypes throughout the ages.

It is not a question of the right or wrong of the ideas. If they are wrong, then the dissenters, who are in the majority, have no reason to fear them. Simple explanation of their fundamental error would be sufficient to render them powerless and futile. If they are sometimes right (as the ideas of Bruno or Galileo were progressive and right), then give all a chance to hear the truth, and to accept or reject it.

Only the man with a conscious or unconscious doubt of his position, especially if he is on the side of the majority, needs feel called upon to suppress an unpopular opinion and persecute the one who expresses such an opinion. The really superior person, who is intellectually sure of his ground, will be content to use the cultural weapons of discussion and reason in attempting to detect error from truth.

Another, although less vicious, example of the

individual who secures gratification in the misfortune of someone else, is afforded in the busybody type of person who goes around his or her circle of acquaintances bringing the latest news of adversity that has befallen someone. Notwithstanding the open expressions of sympathy that are vented, the eagerness with which the oracle unfolds his story of somebody's troubles carries a connotation of pleasure which a little psychologic insight readily perceives. A very primitive Unconscious is being gratified. Every small town has its particular citizen who is especially known for his untiring energy in heralding the details of calamity. He (or she) is frequently the chief unofficial mourner at every local funeral. This is a phase of "Main Street" culture which happens to be a characteristic expression of the Caveman.

Wit is a diverting short-cut from the stiffness and restrictions so constantly demanded by the conventions of social life. The whole evolution of civilization has been the history of repressing primitive instincts. With this constant repression and inhibition, there develops within us a tension of greater or lesser degree. The constant tendency of the elementary side of our nature is to relieve this tension. And anything that contributes to this form of relaxation is a mental and physical tonic. Of course, an excess of tonic, like an excess of any good thing, is undesirable.

*Humor and Adolescence*

Besides wit, petty mischief offers a favorite outlet to the youth and adolescent. It is the unconscious prompting and striving for some vague, indefinite goal of satisfaction which makes gang-companionship, with all its evil potentialities, so alluring to the boy entering upon the age of puberty.

Practical adolescent psychology has taught us that a substitute form of gratification for the destructive tendencies of the gang can be obtained by the youth in athletic contests, country hikes, woodcraft, and other diversions that afford a means of getting "back to nature" in its best sense. These activities offer a healthy, constructive outlet for the pent-up psychic steam that accumulates so rapidly during the critical period of the boy's life when he is undergoing profound physical and psychological changes.

Wit and humor are strikingly in evidence during the adolescent period. As an instance of the development of this faculty, it is generally conceded that the leading college comic papers, conducted entirely by youths, many quite inexperienced, contain better examples of real, spontaneous wit and humor than the national comic publications which have a nation-wide field of professional "humorists" to draw from.

The psychology of wit takes into consideration

the intellectual standard of both speaker and listeners. Subtle jokes that find appreciation in persons of keen mind go over the heads of those with less perception. This tendency is often observed in vaudeville audiences, which are apt to comprise people of all types and degrees of intellectual development. A particularly subtle joke is told by the performer, and here and there an individual in the audience will "get it." A few seconds later quite a large number will begin to snicker, and finally the balance of the audience will start to laugh—for the most part because they have caught the spirit of the occasion, even if they have missed the point made by the comedian.

### Jokes and Ancient Taboos

Those who have gone deeply into the study of primitive tribes have enabled us to see the significance underlying the universal mother-in-law jokes. Primitive races have formulated elaborate systems of taboos, and none is more important than that governing the conduct and relations between mother-in-law and son-in-law.

The psychological explanation of this is that the son-in-law sees in his wife's mother certain traits which caused him to fall in love with his wife, so that there is an emotional response to many of the mother-in-law's actions or expressions. These are unconsciously, rather than consciously, noted, however, and on the part of the mother-in-law, there is the ambivalent feeling of tenderness and hostility toward her daughter's husband. The tenderness is an unconscious reciprocation of the young man's favorable notice of her personal qualites. The hostility is due to a desire, likewise unconscious, to protect herself against infatuation with the new, and often attractive, addition to the family circle. The affection of mother-in-law for son-in-law is not by any means uncommon in the modern world, even if the alleged traditional enmity is more advertised and forms the motive for most of the jokes. In any event, the situation is very involved psychologically, and has received even more attention in a serious way from the ancients than from ourselves in the jocular.

Among people of little cultural development, wit becomes less and less subtle and descends to a correspondingly lower intellectual scale. Persons under the influence of alcohol, that is, where the conscious inhibitions are partially removed, may consider a lewd remark as quite humorous.

As in dreams, sex and ego, either subtle or obvious, form the underlying themes of most jokes. So either of these tendencies may readily veer into the questionable through the force of their native impulse, especially when the conscious repressions are relaxed by convivial associations or the influence of Bacchus. Freud has summed it up in these words: "Under the influence of alcohol the adult again becomes a child who derives pleasure from the free disposal of his mental stream without being restricted by the pressure of logic.''

The sexual undercurrent, so prevalent in jokes, is indicated to an extent by the great amount of cynical wit directed against the institution of marriage. The fundamental reason for this is the ever-present contrast between the primitive sexual urge of man and the monogamic restrictions which are formally prescribed by society. That they have been, and are, so widely honored in the breach, is another thing. Shaw touched on this theme with his characteristic incisive wit when he said in effect that man is fascinated by marriage because it combines the maximum of temptation with the minimum of opportunity.

An example of the way a joke, based on the sexual motive, may achieve a wide popularity is afforded in the expressive term ''Cleopold,'' which had acquired some vogue in the smart circles of Europe. This appellation was given by a wit to the late King Leopold of Belgium on account of his attentions to the French dancer, Cleo. This also offers an illustration of what is known as condensation; combining syllables from two different words into one word, giving it a harmonious sound, and a *naïve* meaning.

Jokes, which by indirection, enable a wit to turn a promising situation into one of disparagement to others, are often very effective, sometimes crushing. The following incident may be mentioned to illustrate this: Two speculating business

men, by a risky venture, amassed an enormous
fortune and determined to force their way into
high society. Among other things, they had their
portraits painted by a noted artist. The costly
pictures were exhibited for the first time at a
large gathering, and the hosts themselves accompanied a prominent art critic to the wall on which
the portraits hung side by side, in order to evoke
from him a favorable criticism. After carefully
examining the pictures for some time, he appeared
to be puzzled, as if something were missing.
Finally, pointing to the bare space between the
portraits, he asked: "And where is the Savior?"

### Wit and Laughter

The natural sequel of wit or a joke is to laugh.
We have all had the almost unbearable experience
wherein our sense of humor had been struck very
pronouncedly, but the proprieties of the occasion
made it imperative that we should not give way
visibly or audibly to our feelings.

As a consequence, we have had the painful sensation of being choked up with something that
should come out, or express itself. Thus, we were
under a nerve-racking tension, quite ready, as we
say, to "explode." Laughter is the physical manifestation which accompanies the response to the
stimuli of wit, jokes and humor generally. It is
the means of a free and quick discharge of psychic
energy.

Besides the common variety of good-natured wit, there is also the well-known type of wit which causes pain or embarrassment to the person at whom the shaft of witticism is aimed. The perpetrator of this kind of joke, thus exhibits a strong current of sadism, which is present in all of us, but in widely varying degrees. One causes another pain and gets satisfaction out of it. And as it is done as a "joke," he does not feel the onus of committing a deliberate anti-social act. "It was only a joke." It is axiomatic that this type of individual seldom appreciates a joke that is on himself. His sadist characteristics are too dominating.

Persons who good-naturedly laugh at or pass off jokes of this kind on themselves are evidencing a well-defined masochistic quality, which is also inherent in everyone.

The so-called "practical jokes," in particular, are frequently of an irritating or even destructive character. The unconscious mind is fundamentally primitive and uncultured, and takes a positive delight in causing pain to others. It craves excitement. The conscious mind, governed more by social influences, does much to offset the primitive desires. It is notable in people whose altruistic or social qualities have had little opportunity to develop—i.e. who are largely under the influence of their primitive nature, and especially so among savages—that they take a weird satisfaction in the sight of painful experience of others.

Atavistic traits are universal, even among civilized people, and are brought to the surface most pronouncedly in times of war, thus affording an opportunity for the psychic and physical gratification of the archaic qualities of the Cave-creature within us.

I have elaborated on wit, humor and jokes as characteristic diversions of the Caveman, because of their importance in this rôle, and their constant usage because of ready accessibility. A number of other favorites could be analysed in detail if space permitted. Amusement in general, with which wit, humor and jokes are intimately associated, has many interesting angles as means of relieving the psychic tension.

### Adventure and Physical Endeavor

In play, sports and athletic contests, we permit ourselves to live over again, in a healthy, constructive way, our remote biological past. This form of diversion not only exercises the muscles, but is valuable as a means of promoting the vital functions of the ductless glands and autonomic nervous system, which are so closely interrelated with our emotions and primitive nature—the mechanism which prepares us for flight or fight in times of danger. In healthy athletic pastimes, we are sublimating this energy and the primitive emotions into a socially acceptable channel.

Travel and adventure also are forms of diversion that satisfy a craving. Man has some deeply inlaid nomadic tendencies, and travel enables those with the means to indulge this form of recreation, to forget for a time the grind of organized routine life. The same urge (when not strictly economic) lies behind the wealthy tourist, traveling in luxury, and the penniless hobo, riding in his "side-door Pullman." Each gratifies a primitive desire to flee from reality—the treadmill of concentrated effort—in a manner that conforms to his means, imagination and training.

Adventure! What romances, novels, yes, human histories, have been written around this great subject. Every normal boy and girl is embued with the spirit of adventure. It is the beckoning will-o'-the-wisp which lies beyond the portals of the present. It lures us on and on in our day dreams from the commonplace of our environment to the unrealized and unrealizable phantasies we associate with the future. The interest of many readers of sensational fiction is due to the fact that they identify themselves with the hero, live with him through a series of absorbing adventures, and fall in love with the heroine, who lives happily ever after. Female readers, of course, identify themselves with the heroine and her exploits.

We have observed how youth is restless, energetic, craving action, and sidestepping laborious duties. The call of adventure is the most romantic of all diversions and the most difficult to satisfy, because of its unlimited, indefinite scope. For most of us, it always lies beyond—like the El-dorado of old. It is this spirit, in part, which makes the played-up glamour of war so attractive to youth. The glamour imagined is that associated with wars in earlier history, which has been idealized by the passing of time, and not the deadly monotonous routine of modern war, which is a gigantic technological mechanism.

It is the *spirit* of adventure, however, which we are discussing, and the primitive attraction of war to youth led William James to suggest the possibility of a moral substitute for war, by diverting this archaic craving to other channels of large physical action, such as life on sea, adventurous diversions, and even work at hazardous occupations, such as in mines, or in great engineering projects.

### BIBLIOGRAPHY

FREUD, SIGMUND, *Wit and its Relation to the Unconscious*, New York, 1917.
BERGSON, HENRI, *Laughter*, New York, 1914.
BAIN, A., *The Emotions and the Will*, 2nd Ed., 1865.
LIPPS, THEODOR, *Comic and Humor*, 1898.
SPENCER, HERBERT, *Psychology of Laughter*, London, 1881.
SIDIS, BORIS, *Psychology of Laughter*, New York, 1913.
TRIDON, ANDRÉ, *Psycho-analysis, its History, Theory and Practice*, Chapter, IX, New York, 1919.
EASTMAN, MAX, *The Sense of Humor*, New York, 1921.

# CHAPTER VI

## THE CAVEMAN'S TRICKS

My soul is sailing through the sea,
But the Past is heavy and hindereth me.
The Past hath crusted cumbrous shells
That hold the flesh of cold sea-swells
About my soul.
—SIDNEY LANIER, *Barnacles*.

IT is often annoying to have tricks played on us. It is doubly annoying when we play tricks on ourselves—that is, when the deep, underlying personality within us—the Unconscious—gets the upper hand in a most vexatious way and completely outwits our rational self. Most of these little tricks are so commonplace and recur so constantly in one way or another that we dismiss the incidents without further reflection. Occasionally, they are extremely provoking and positively embarrassing if they expose to others what appears to be our weakness or a failing.

Why is it that we forget certain things, particularly when we are most anxious to remember them, or when we think we are especially desirous of remembering them? In a way we wish to remember them; in another way, a more fundamental, more primitive way, we wish to forget them. We cannot dismiss the fact that there is

117

a dual character which has disguised itself in the form of a single physical entity. Things are not what they seem. We look at an individual and see a single face, a single person. We have overlooked the fact, evidenced by centuries-old proof, and now scientifically confirmed, that every human face is a Janus-face; every person a dual personality.

The more clearly this is realized, the more safe and sane we will be in our actions, the more consistent and ethical in our social relations, and the happier in our own little spheres. When people had no inkling of the innermost operations of their psychic and physical being, they burned men and women as sorcerers and witches who acted irrationally—or at least, too conspicuously so. They felt an irresistible force within themselves that was somewhat out of control of their conscious faculties, and they suspected everyone else who showed signs of "queerness" of having the same quality, very highly magnified. They were correct in assuming that, to all intents and purposes, another energetic factor existed— one that functioned without the conscious will— but they were wrong in conceiving it to be of an extraneous character. It was, in fact, an inseparable component of their complete personality.

### Forgetfulness

Forgetfulness is perhaps the most universal of our self-irritating shortcomings. We are always forgetting things that we meant to do. We are forever overlooking little duties we intended to perform. It has been noticed by some observing persons that we are more apt to forget certain kinds of duties than others. Why? Has the memory cultivated a sense of discrimination? Does it pick and choose among the various obligations imposed upon it?

That portion of our psychic stream known as the Unconscious—the will-force of the Caveman—is purely egotistic and very discriminating in its likes, which are always of the free-and-easy, the pleasant, the exhilarating type. Its process of accomplishing the desired result is by a method termed "repression." Things that have an unpleasant connotation to the Unconscious are repressed, or "forgotten." The more primitive the individual is, the more obviously this force works. The more intellectual one is, the more subtly it functions. Often it is quite uncanny in its *modus operandi*. Memories that are unpleasant to the Unconscious, and associations which would tend to recall them, are repressed out of the Conscious. They are held down into the immense reservoir of the Unconscious. For the convenience of everyday life, we say they are *forgotten*.

There are some things we can never forget; some we rarely forget; others we are very prone to forget. As a general rule, we tend to forget those things which are offensive to our ego, or which would deprive us of a pleasure. We tend to remember those incidents in our experience which are satisfying to our ego, and which give us a pleasurable, exhilarating sensation or feeling of well-being.

Darwin was not a psychologist, much less a Freudian, but in his autobiography he wrote: "I had, during many years, followed a golden rule, namely, that whenever a published fact, a new observation or thought came across me, which was opposed to my general results, to make a memorandum of it without fail and at once; for I found by experience that such facts and thoughts were far more apt to escape from the memory than favourable ones."

Notwithstanding the rare intellectual powers and rational development of Darwin, which assured a conscious desire to remember unfavourable testimony, criticism and inner doubts, his unconscious mind, the unregenerate ego, was in the long run triumphant and repressed the things that were objectionable to its whims.

It has been noted universally that we are more apt to mislay a bill than a check; more apt to forget to mail a check than a bill. If a letter is entrusted to us for mailing, we accept the obligation as a matter of courtesy, even if we often forget to place it in the letter box until several days later. There is nothing particularly exhilarating to the ego in mailing the letter of a friend or acquaintance, or even a commonplace letter of our own. If we start out intending to post a love letter we have written, there is good assurance of one hundred per cent. efficiency of our memory.

Dr. Ernest Jones mentions that he once allowed a letter to lie on his writing desk several days for reasons quite unknown. Finally he mailed it, but it was returned from the dead letter office, as he had forgotten to address it. After he had addressed it, he took it to the post office, but this time without a stamp. At this point, he had to admit to himself his aversion against sending the letter at all.

I recently observed a convincing incident of this kind, although the party in question did not think of the unconscious motive until I had called it to his attention. The assistant to the head of an important bookkeeping office told me that he had just dropped a letter in the mail box without a stamp. I suggested there must have been a reason why he did not wish the letter to reach the addressée. He replied that, on the contrary, he was especially anxious to have it go out properly and for that reason had dropped the letter in the box himself, instead of having a boy mail it. Admitting that his intentions were the best, I insisted there was an unconscious reason why he did not want the letter to be delivered. With a bland smile, he stated that, as a matter of fact, the letter contained some information which in his judgment should not have been given, but that he had been directed to send it by his superior, and he had taken special pains to note on his memoranda papers that he had been so authorized, to protect himself from future criticism.

Some examples of forgetfulness show considerable unconscious ingenuity, either in thwarting a conscious desire, or sometimes in assisting our conscious mind to accomplish its purpose. A. E. Maeder has cited an excellent illustration of the latter. A house surgeon had an appointment in town, but was denied the privilege of leaving the hospital until his chief, who was filling a dinner engagement, should return later in the evening. As his appointment was important, he decided to disregard the instructions of his superior and go to town. When he returned later, he found to his astonishment that he had left the light burning in his room, which he had never done before in the two years he had occupied the room. A little reflection made clear to him the unconscious motive in doing this. His superior in passing the window on the way to his own home would see the light burning and take for granted that the house surgeon was within. The unconscious mind had intuitively sized up a situation which had altogether escaped the attention of the conscious mind, and decreed that the light should be overlooked.

### The Ego and Names

A very common difficulty is in remembering names. We meet a person, are introduced, and the name seems to escape us immediately after the sound echoes mockingly in our ears. This tendency is widely varied among different people, and it is rarely a question of intelligence or "memory" in the usual sense of that term. I have a friend of exceptional intelligence, very effective in argument, which he is able to sustain with unlimited facts for which he has a phenomenal memory. His knowledge covers a wide range of the social sciences, economics and theology. However, he seems absolutely unable to retain the name of a person whom he has met for the first time, or even several times.

Dickens and other celebrities have remarked on their poor memory for names. Their ego, absolutely under unconscious influences, for which they were in no way consciously responsible, attempted to ignore certain individuals—possible competitors for fame—by repressing their identity out of consciousness, "forgetting" them—or to put it more crudely and bluntly, to deny their existence.

Names and persons have a most intimate reaction on our psyche. When we meet an individual, we may express our pleasure (real or assumed) and greet him civilly, in accordance with the conventions. The ego, however, is not essentially civil. It is suspicious of strangers, either unconsciously fears, distrusts or dislikes them, and in order to eliminate them from its little world, it represses the fact of their existence. The shortness of one's memory for names is in inverse measure of the power of one's ego. If the name is similar to or identical with our own, it is adding insult to injury according to the primitive notion of the Unconscious. It represents an infringement on our personality. Our name is very near and dear to us. Along comes a personality bearing a label like our own. To the ego, this is unfair competition, an unwarranted affront. If we do not forget the name in so unusual a case, our unconscious antipathy is very often reflected by a conscious aversion or dislike for the unsuspecting offender. Those who have some knowledge of the operations of their psychic mechanism understand this situation and are not agitated by it. The great majority of people say: "There is something about him I don't like. I distrust him." After this prejudice is worn away by the mollifying influence of time, they may become intimate friends.

### Mislaying Objects

An exasperating annoyance which every individual is the victim of at times is the mislaying of objects and being unable to locate them when wanted, until they come to notice by accident or through some association of ideas. Sometimes a chain of associations that is quite obvious will recall the location of a misplaced article. At other times the association is so subtle that it escapes our conscious mental processes altogether.

A most perfect example of the latter is given by Freud in his *General Introduction to Psychoanalysis*. A young man told Freud that a few years previously a misunderstanding arose in his married life. He felt his wife was too cool and even though he willingly acknowledged her excellent qualities, they lived without any tenderness between them. One day she brought him a book which she had thought might interest him. He thanked her for this attention, promised to read the book, put it in a handy place and could not find it again. Several months passed, during which he occasionally remembered the mislaid book and tried in vain to find it. About half a year later his mother, who lived a distance from them, fell ill. His wife left the house in order to nurse her mother-in-law. The condition of the patient became serious, and gave his wife an opportunity of showing her best side. One evening he came home filled with enthusiasm and gratitude toward his wife for her devotion to his mother. He approached his writing desk, opened a certain drawer with no definite intention but as if with somnambulistic certainty, and the first thing he found was the book so long mislaid.

With the cessation of the unconscious motive to keep the book hidden, his inability to find it also came to an end. Similar cases, though less romantic in their complications, are numerous. Persons lose objects when they have fallen out with their donors and no longer wish to be reminded of them. Objects also may be lost if one no longer likes the things themselves and wants to supply oneself with a pretext for substituting other and more desirable things in their stead.

There is a close relation between this type of unconscious motive and in letting a thing fall and break—"accidentally on purpose," as the old saying goes, which is an unwitting observation containing an element of truth. The same intention toward the object is shown. A strongly sadistic individual would be apt to indulge in the latter method more frequently than one in whom the masochistic tendencies predominate. Breaking and destroying things are a symbolical form of sadism. Many accidents attributed to carelessness are the result of unconscious, disguised wishes that the accident would happen. Carelessness, as a matter of fact, is the absence of the conscious wish.

The objection is likely to be raised that this method of reasoning attributes to the unconscious mind powers that are too sweeping, and without warrant. It may be difficult at the outset to accept the conclusion that the Unconscious really registers an impression of all our visual, auditory and other sensory experiences. However, there is an abundance of evidence that tends to confirm it. The far greater part of this accumulation of impressions is never reproduced or projected into consciousness, at least in a recognizable form. But when all the evidence in the case is carefully weighed and the facts analyzed, we can accept no other conclusion than that of the limitless, ineradicable memory of our Unconscious.

## Unconscious Memories

Many examples could be offered to substantiate this contention. Perhaps no better illustration can be given of the ability of the mind unconsciously to absorb and reproduce sensations (auditory in this instance) than that quoted by Coleridge in his *Biographia Literaria* of the illiterate German girl ill with fever, who talked at great length in the classic languages. It is suggestive enough to bear repetition here:

"In a Roman Catholic town in Germany, a young woman, who could neither read nor write, was seized with a fever, and was said by the priests to be possessed of a devil, because she was heard talking Latin, Greek and Hebrew. Whole sheets of her ravings were written out, and found to consist of sentences intelligible in themselves, but having slight connection with each other. Of her Hebrew sayings, only a few could be traced to the Bible, and most of them seemed to be in the Rabbinical dialect. All trick was out of the question; the woman was a simple creature; there was no doubt as to the fever . . . At last the mystery was unveiled by a physician, who determined to trace back the girl's history, and who, after much trouble, discovered that at the age of nine she had been charitably taken by an old Protestant pastor, a great Hebrew scholar, in whose house she lived till his death. On further inquiry, it appeared to have been the old man's custom for years to walk up and down a passage of his house into which the kitchen opened, and to read to himself with a loud voice out of his books. The books were ransacked, and among them were found several of the Greek and Latin Fathers, together with a collection of Rabbinical writings. In these works, so many of the passages taken down at the young woman's bedside were identified, that there could be no reasonable doubt as to their source.''

It is a commonplace that people who are out of their mind from fever, injury or other misfortune—when the inhibitory faculty of consciousness is removed—will say things that quite obviously had been consciously forgotten, and very likely that they must have wished to forget, as often the grosser and more primitive side of the personality is exposed in these instances.

The capacity of the unconscious mind for reproducing "forgotten" impressions, and even impressions that were never consciously noted, is so vast and far-reaching in its effects that we cannot begin to fathom its possibilities. Besides the commonplace tendencies that continually find expression, there are unusual evidences of unconscious mental activity which are puzzling in the extreme. Among a few of the means that emphasize the unconscious psychic processes are hypnotism, somnambulism, automatic writing, crystal gazing, etc., and there is no telling how many of the phenomena that pass as spiritism, and telepathy, or thought transmission, are purely products of this vast field. Auto-suggestion, visions, various faith cures, and numerous other features that have been associated with various religious and ethical cults, are from evidence of the facts at hand, among the manifestations of the Unconscious.

Maeterlinck, in one of his works, gives an account of a girl who was hypnotized and whose memory was forced back to earliest childhood, then to infancy, and finally to a supposedly prenatal state. According to this account, the timbre of the girl's voice suddenly changed and became that of an old woman who claimed that she had lived at a certain period prior to the girl's birth. Pursuing further the method of regression, the timbre of the voice changed once more and became that of an old man, who claimed to have been a soldier of the Guards of the first Napoleon. Demonstrations of this kind are accepted by some persons as proof of reincarnation. Before we accept such conclusions, however, it is well to consider the capacity of the unconscious mind for utilizing scraps of its inexhaustible supply of material, piecing them together and reproducing them in a fantastic drama such as only could be conceived in that fertile field. The common tendency of dreams and hallucinations is also along this channel of grotesque reproduction of recent or old and "forgotten" experiences.

Our aimless scribbles while we wait with pencil in hand at the telephone, or when otherwise disengaged from directed mental effort, reveal peculiarities of our inner self that we seldom consciously recognize. We all express our unconscious desires, attitudes and thoughts, usually unrecognizable, when we find ourselves with pencil and paper and without anything definite to write. Artists, skilled in the technique of their craft, have been known to draw very elaborate and grotesque pictures while under the influence of the Unconscious. Nor is it rare for people to write at some length, solely from unconscious dictation. All writing is a more or less combined product of the conscious and unconscious mental processes. The Unconscious, when coördinated with directed mental effort is the fountainhead of creative inspiration.

## Erroneous Actions and Speech

Slips of the tongue are governed by a very positive attitude of the unconscious mind. If we consciously take the greatest pains to protect ourselves from making an oral mistake and then say the opposite to what we consciously desired to express, the fact that there is an underlying wish should be quite obvious. That the import of

tongue slips is essentially in accord with our unconscious wishes is evidenced by the fact that we
seldom notice them (and our unconscious mind is
intuitively alert), although we always notice them
in others.

Every one in his daily routine is obliged to do
many things and carry out instructions that are
not entirely pleasing to the ego, even though they
are not consciously questioned. It is in fulfilling
these obligations, and in conforming to the requirements of common courtesy and tactfulness
that we are apt to leave out a word, a prefix or
syllable, or put one in when it should be left out,
and thereby convey a meaning the opposite to
that which we intended to express. There is inevitably a wish or aversion at the bottom of these
little sins of omission and commission, although
it may at times be buried so deeply as to be difficult to recognize the fact.

The unconscious motives in these instances are
so palpably based on the egotistical, primitive,
selfish desires that we do not care to recognize
them as our own inner thoughts. When a physician said to his prosperous patient, "I hope you
will not be able to leave your bed soon," he unconsciously wanted to hold on to this professional
meal-ticket, even though his conscious ideals and
ethics were unquestioned.

The conceited lecturer who said "those who
understand this subject can be counted on one
finger—I mean the fingers of one hand," was

unconsciously prompted by his ego to pay himself a little tribute.

Mistakes in writing have the same psychological basis as slips of the tongue, with the qualification that omissions of words and letters seem to indicate a distaste for writing and an impatience to get through with it. Even among those not averse to writing, however, the tendency to use terms contradictory to our conscious will is common.

Erroneous actions that are so often dismissed without second thought, as being due to absent-mindedness, are particularly good examples of unconscious wishes linked up with some associations of comfort or well-being. Physicians have noticed that when reaching the house of a patient, where they felt especially at home, they were apt to take out of their pocket the key to their own door and only upon reflection finally ring the bell.

People never hum aimless tunes. The tune selected, or the words to which it has been set, will be found to have a direct or indirect bearing upon the individual's thoughts or general attitude at the time. Pfister has collected several interesting illustrations on this subject.

Aside from our intellectual self which is characterized by conscious and directed thought, there is another force at work within us, always active and struggling for expression. This is our primitive self, which functions through our unconscious actions and undirected, intuitive thought.

## BIBLIOGRAPHY

PFISTER, OSKAR, *The Psychoanalytic Method,* New York, 1917.

LAY, WILFRID, *Man's Unconscious Conflict,* New York, 1917.

PUTNAM, J. J., *Human Motives,* Boston, 1915.

JAMES, WILLIAM, *Psychology,* Vols. I and II, New York.

FREUD, SIGMUND, *Psychopathology of Everyday Life,* New York, 1914.

FREUD, SIGMUND, *General Introduction to Psychoanalysis,* New York, 1920.

# CHAPTER VII

## THE CAVEMAN'S PASSION

Everyone bears within him an image of a woman, inherited from his mother; it determines his attitude toward women as a whole, whether to honour, despise, or remain generally indifferent to them.—FREDERICK NIETZSCHE.

THE substream of our unconscious mind is a deep and mighty current, over the surface of which there is spread a shallow coverlet, completely disguising the unfathomable depths below. The disguise is normally complete to ourselves, as well as to others. Having penetrated the surface, the deeper we go into the substream, the more astounding are the disclosures brought to light. And we can never go deep enough not to find new wonders, new sensations, new revelations.

Of all the factors comprising our Unconscious, none are more subtle, and at the same time more potent and far-reaching, than those contributing to our erotic disposition, our love-life—the Caveman's passion.

There is a clear distinction between the elements entering into our conscious love and those that compose the basic, unconscious urge. The latter are the deeply ingrained, far-reaching biological factors that we have inherited from untold generations in the evolution of the race. These are the crassly sexual qualities whose innermost promptings and expressions have given rise to prudery, as an attempt to over-sublimate them by suppression as a form of compensation, rather than to control them.

The conscious elements are the idealistic properties that are acquired with the rounding out of our cultural development, combining affection, esteem, admiration, respect.

It stands to reason that a healthy, happy, adaptable human being must adjust himself or herself so that these two erotic streams are coordinated, each interacting upon the other, and obtaining normal expression in a socially acceptable manner. If the attempt is made to deny or frustrate the more primitive of these urges, the road is being paved for their outbreak in abnormal channels.

Throughout the whole realm of nature, the chief end of life is to make one sex attractive to, and attracted by, the other sex. The manifestations of this principle, while more open and undisguised among animals than among mankind, are nevertheless just as pronounced in the latter as in the former. Even in the vegetable world, the same elaborate scheme is evidenced by nature on every point—although there is a total lack of awareness on the part of the agencies involved—to bring together in manifold, ingenious ways the two elements that are essential to propagation.

The unending expression of sex phenomena in all its variations and disguises rivals that of economic determinism in influencing the drama of life. The two great urges whose impelling power dominates our life are physical hunger (the craving for material subsistence) and spiritual hunger (the yearning for love).

In every normal individual there is an unconscious thrill, sometimes consciously perceived, upon sight of an attractive person of the opposite sex. More often the reaction of this phenomenon never rises to consciousness, as in facing the demands of reality, we cannot concern ourselves with every passing object that pleases our erotic Unconscious. Nevertheless, the unconscious thrill is invariably present, and we often consciously reflect it by casting a second glance or manifesting some other form of sexual interest which we may not care to recognize as such.

While this unconscious trait of our psyche is not very discriminating, reacting to all fairly attractive members of the opposite sex, there is another feature of our unconscious erotic mechanism that evidences a marked discrimination.

This factor in our psychic make-up is loaded with possibilities for making or marring our prospects of happiness. It is an unconscious instrumentality that tends to direct us with irresistible force toward an unknown goal. It is responsible for countless marital failures, ruined lives, infidelity, divorce. While it cannot be obliterated or suppressed, an understanding of its method of operation might have saved a large percentage of unhappy marriages from their ultimate wreckage, or prevented in the first place the union that could end only in disaster.

What is the unconscious influence that causes us instinctively to take to, or show a preference for, a certain type of individual of the opposite sex? Why is it that some people fall in love at first sight—if only to fall out again as soon as they get a chance to become acquainted? This influence is so subtle in its operation that we seldom stop to realize that there are types to which we are attracted, others to which we remain indifferent, and still others that we are repelled by.

The attraction of one sex for the other is one of the great fundamental principles of life—in all forms of life. Nature has devised elaborate mechanisms to work toward this end. And it might be emphasized that nature takes no account of the social conventions and cultural demands of civilization. It is the very important, practical job of the people who compose modern society to make some harmonious adjustment between their innate biological urges and the social requirements.

## The Parent Image

There is one particular pivotal point in the mechanism of sex attraction, which constitutes nature's powerful but undiscriminating device for carrying out the biological plan. In every male infant, from the moment of its earliest impressions, there begins to form a mental image of a woman—normally the mother, or her substitute, nurse, grandmother, aunt, elder sister or other female who may be intimately concerned with the task of nourishing and catering to the wants of the infant. The female child is similarly influenced by the father image—which may substitute the brother, grandfather or other male relative.

The character of this image in the psyche of the individual governs his future attitude toward those of the opposite sex. Its normal characteristic is flexibility and adaptation, and like all other human qualities, it should develop and run its course. Its chief function is to act as an unconscious or instinctive guide in enabling us readily to determine our preferences in the sexual or love object. This picture is carried around in our psyche, and a comparison is unconsciously made whenever we see one of the opposite sex that interests us. We never lose it, although in normal human beings, as puberty is approached, the image becomes weaned from its first exclusive attraction.

The abnormal course that is open as an alternative results in the parent image's becoming static. Instead of the unconscious image's being transferred from its specific infantile object and acting as a general guide, it remains fixed on its original, primitive goal, and consequently warps the individual's outlook on life.

In almost every instance, it will be observed that intelligent and otherwise eligible women who remain unmarried through life, or until comparatively late in life, are the daughters of men of commanding personality, such as would be apt to wield a powerful influence on the imagination of their daughters. Following the same rule, most bachelors I have known have been the sons of women of impressive or outstanding personality. The parent of mediocre or insignificant personality is much less apt to sway the unconscious mind of the son or daughter for an extended period after adolescence.

The more obvious effect of the crystallization of this image is to instigate intense conflicts which the conscious mind attempts to repress, and therefore vast amounts of energy are wasted in the resultant mental struggle. The ancients, without realizing the cause of this situation, were profoundly impressed by its effects, as we can today observe by reading their literature. The drama of King Œdipus, in its several variations by the foremost Greek poets—Sophocles and Euripides, especially—is the most striking example in all literature—classic or modern. This tragedy of Œdipus, who was impelled by his fate to kill his father and unknowingly win his mother for a wife, led to the adoption of the name of its principle as a term particularly suited to express the situation.

That Œdipus felt intensely the conflict which beset him is clear in the following words from Sophocles' version:

"Am I not by nature a villain? If I must needs flee the country, and having fled am to be permitted neither to behold mine own, nor to set foot on my native soil; or I am doomed to be yoked in wedlock to my mother, and to kill outright my father Polybus, who reared, who begot me. And would not anyone, pronouncing all this to be the work of a ruthless demon upon me, be right in his words? Then O may I never, may I never, thou spotless majesty of heaven, see this day, but may I be gone from among mankind into darkness ere that I view such a taint of misery come upon me."

Equally illuminating is Jocasta's understanding of mankind's unconscious incestuous promptings, as evidenced by her reply: "But have thou no fear of the bridal alliance with thy mother; for many among mankind have ere now, and that in dreams, done incest with a mother; but whomsoever this reckons as nothing, he bears his life the easiest."

While the early Greeks, and later philosophers, have shown that they had recognized the potency of the parent fixation, it remained for Freud to develop the hypothesis along scientific lines.

The real analogy of the Œdipus tragedy to the

ordinary parent fixation is a spiritual one. In ignorance, Œdipus married his mother, Jocasta, who bore him several children. In ignorance of the mother-image which dominates him, the subject-type under discussion marries in effect this symbolical image, rather than a living being. And as disaster befell the incestuous alliance of Œdipus and Jocasta, so misfortune falls to the lot of the man who mates spiritually with the mother-image. In each case the character of the avenging Nemesis was originally mysterious and unknown. Finally, the oracle revealed the situation in the mythological drama; and it has fallen to the lot of psychological science to play the rôle of the modern oracle and point out the origin of the affliction and the possibilities for remedying it. Otto Rank has offered a constructive suggestion in these words: "The detachment of the growing individual from the authority of the parents is one of the most necessary, but also one of the most painful achievements of evolution. It is absolutely necessary for this detachment to take place."

A popular misconception has arisen of the Freudian attitude regarding the question of incestuous ideas. By pointing out the evidence that these phenomena exist, and noting their influence, disguised by symbolism, on mankind, the analysts are not "advocating" incestuous thoughts, either unconscious or conscious, but are merely recognizing a condition. It is considered that the

general incredulity of the normal grown-up man
to the significance of incest wishes is due to the
man's aversion of his own former wishes of this
type, which have since succumbed to repression.

It has been found that a man tends to marry a
woman who bears some resemblance to his mother.
There is no limit to the points of resemblance, real
or imaginary (as they sometimes are), that the
man may find in the object of his love, which the
Unconscious perceives as likening to the mother,
from whom it has received so many comforts. The
likeness may be extremely slight, something about
the hair, the walk, an attitude, or, perhaps more
frequently, a resemblance in point of figure. Then
again, it may be entirely imaginary, a phantom
which the Unconscious, in its crude, primitive
manner, has conjured into reality.

But there is often a tangible resemblance.
Years ago, Karl Pearson was puzzled to find that
the color of eyes was more alike in man and wife
than it should be in first cousins, according to
biological theory.  As a man tends to marry a
woman resembling his mother, and a woman tends
to marry a man resembling her father, the color
of the eyes must be among the first of all like-
nesses to be recognized and seized upon by the
Unconscious.  As the percentage of men who have
inherited the color of eyes of their mother, and
women the color of eyes of their father, is very
great, it explains the reason for this point of common resemblance between husband and wife.

There can be no doubt but what there are still important principles of heredity to be discovered. It is quite possible that some of these secrets of nature may govern the transmission of characteristics from parent to child of the opposite sex, as a means of furthering the scheme of life.

Normal or common traits are more difficult to trace for obvious reasons. Abnormal and unusual traits are easier to observe. One instance of this kind is the ocular defect known as Daltonism or color-blindness. A color-blind man usually will not have color-blind children; nor will the children of his sons be color-blind, but the sons of his daughters will be color-blind. This form of ocular abnormality is rare in women, but it is transmitted from man to grandson through the *female* line. Color-blindness is understood to have its seat, not in the visual center, but in the eye itself, or in the nerves of the eye, whereby imperfect sensations are transmitted to the brain. Hæmophilia, or the "bleeding disease," a more serious affliction, has the same hereditary characteristics.

## A Neurotic Basis

The individual who carries the parent image in his Unconscious so that it dominates his actions is a typical neurotic. This image is present in everyone, and it always exerts more or less influence, but in the normal person it is not a dominating factor.

The presence of the mother image does not imply that the picture is a replica of the mother as she appears in the adult life of the son. The impression is as she appeared to the Unconscious of the man or youth in his infancy. The neurotic may treat his mother with scant consideration, display ill-temper and even disrespect, and still be dominated by the infantile image of his mother which he unconsciously holds as a model for all womanhood. It is inevitable that all women who come under his observation fail to measure up to this stereotyped standard. Even the mother in the flesh, as she is at the present time, falls short of the ideal that is registered in his psyche.

It is a symbolical image or distorted memory that he unconsciously worships—a living replica of which he is ever trying to find for his own. It is written in the records of fate that he is doomed to disappointment, because such a thing—the living phantasy of his Unconscious—does not exist.

This is the unrecognized factor that causes many men to remain unmarried throughout life. They are unable to find the non-existent mate they are continually looking for.

Even worse is the fate of the man with a dominating mother-fixation who marries, because he soon discovers that his wife is not the woman he thought she was. It is true she is not, nor could she be. It is not within the province of any woman to fill the bill.

Many who are not confirmed neurotics, but who

have strong tendencies in that direction, feel a similar *something* lacking, an indescribable element in their marriage relations. They realize that the woman they have chosen is a good wife, but there is some misgiving which they feel but cannot definitely place or define. An insight into the real situation would show them that they are simply trying to measure up a very human person with the image of a non-existent ideal.

This knowledge, in ordinary cases, will supply the key to the situation, and lead to a satisfactory reorientation of ideas. It will suggest to persons of this type the futility of trying to find the impossible (which is always a neurotic tendency of getting away from reality). Therefore, if not hopeless or too far gone, they will adjust themselves to actualities, realize that a man should love his wife for her own qualities, and not feel slighted because she lacks some imaginary ones. By doing this, he will be forsaking the infantile attitude of the baby who demands the moon, and cries because he cannot have it. This is essentially what the neurotic is doing.

All of these remarks, of course, apply with equal weight to the female neurotic who is dominated by a father-fixation.

The parent-fixation has been found to be the cause of many cases of impotence—termed psychic impotence—because in the wife, the husband's Unconscious senses a member of the mother-sister class, with whom, on account of the incest barrier, it is impossible to experience the consummation of the sex act. For the same reason, it is the cause of frigid wives. The consequences of this condition may better be realized when we take into consideration the fact that impotence and frigidity are universally recognized as fertile breeding grounds for marital disharmony with all its resultant evils.

It has been observed that men of this type who are impotent with their wives, may resort to prostitutes and secure sexual satisfaction. This is because the prostitute, being recognized as a low and fallen woman, is not in the mother-sister class, and therefore the incest barrier in these relations is not operative. The incest barrier, as an hypothesis, has been compared to the incest taboo found among primitive peoples. Its biological reason for existence has been ascribed to an unconscious impediment devised by nature to prevent inbreeding.

### Homosexuality

Homosexuality also has been observed to be a result of a parent fixation. In this case (for men) all women fall under the ban of the incest barrier, and the natural sexual urge is driven into abnormal channels. This perversion leads to the desire for sexual congress with a member of the same sex.

It has thus been found that homosexuality, instead of being due to an inherent trait or vicious character, is conditioned by an unfavorable environment. The boy who is raised in an environment too exclusively feminine or is Mollycoddled beyond all bounds by his mother, may develop into a homosexual.

Where the youth is raised from infancy in a home without the father or other adult male, there is no normal model that the boy can consciously and unconsciously imitate. Being compelled to imitate some one in order to establish a standard of behavior, he copies his mother's attitude of physical indifference to women and physical interest in men. Thus, psychologically, he becomes a woman and as he reaches physical maturity, he will prefer to imagine sexual gratification as a woman would.

The nature of the physiological development of the individual through fetal life and infancy contributes to this result. In the embryonic growth, there is a period when it is neither male nor female, and may later become either one or the other. There is present a rudimentary outline of the physiological characteristics of both sexes. Therefore, when the sex of the fetus is established there are existent certain features of the opposite sex as well. The infant is born with bisexual qualities, traces of which are retained throughout life. The vestigial breasts are noticeable in the male, and hair on the face of the female.

These physical bisexual features are paralleled in the psyche. This is particularly striking in infancy and childhood. There is, for instance, a great deal less difference between little boys and girls mentally than there is between men and women. The early life represents a homosexual stage, with a gradual broadening out toward the heterosexual goal at puberty. However, if the environment is so one-sided that progress toward the heterosexual objective is thwarted, and it may be arrested at any stage of its evolution, then there results a cessation of psychic development at a certain homosexual level.

Bousfield has indicated the evolution of the sexual components of the child in the following manner:[1]

*Infant:* autosexuality ........... 100%
*Child of twelve years of age:*
    Autosexuality ............... 40%
    Homosexuality .............. 50%
    Heterosexuality ............. 10%
*Normal individual at puberty:*
    Autosexuality ............... 20%
    Homosexuality .............. 30%
    Heterosexuality ............. 50%
Any or all of these components may be:
(1) Repressed and then sublimated.
(2) Repressed without adequate sublimation.
        (Causing neuroses, bad habits, etc.)
(3) Not repressed but expressed.
(4) Displaced.

[1] Paul Bousfield, M.D., *The Elements of Practical Psycho-Analysis;* E. P. Dutton & Co., New York.

## Narcissism

That period in the development of the individual which follows the infantile *autosexual,* or *autoerotic,* may best be stressed under the term, *narcissism,* which is so commonly used in the new psychology. It is taken from the well-known Greek mythological character, Narcissus, who fell in love with his own reflection in a pool. Thus enamored of himself, he spurned the approaches of Venus and was destroyed or lost his eyesight, according to the different versions. The virtue of the comparison is that the individual who concentrates *his whole attention* upon himself will perish.

Narcissistic development normally runs its course between the ages of from six to twelve or fourteen, although strong traces of it remain in everyone. It does not represent a conscious self-worship, such as is evidenced in the auto-erotic exhibitionist, but it is more disguised and subtle, and less directly sexual. The child or narcissistic adult considers all things in their relation to himself, and not as related with some other thing or with all other things.

Altogether there is perhaps no tendency that is so rampant in modern life. And its influence reacts on the social relations no less than on the individual. Dr. Smith Ely Jelliffe has stated that the present stage of civilization is chiefly narcissistic. In other words, there is an inertia of social conscience which is directly reflected in the maladjustments of society. We are still at the preadolescent level of social development.

Among the common characteristics of the narcissistic fixation is impatience, the impulse to accomplish something as soon as the wish is conceived. Then, before this may have been even started upon, another infantile desire intrudes itself. And so the wild and futile chase proceeds.

Narcissism of a pronounced type often turns to homosexuality, as it has much of the mechanism of the latter. The modifying condition, however, is that the object admired must be like the individual himself, because in projecting his erotic feelings upon another, he is in effect identifying the second party with himself.

However, if the erotic stream is directed to an heterosexual goal, the love object will in all probability be of a type physically and mentally similar to himself. His own personality is the ideal that others have to measure up to in order to interest him.

### Fetichism

Fetichism is an erotic displacement in which the sex impulse is concentrated upon an object which in itself has no direct erotic significance, but is merely symbolic of the normal sexual aim. It is expressed by seeing or touching a particular part of the body or article of wearing apparel associated with that part of the body. The greatest amount of fetichism seems directed toward the hair, ankles and feet. It is common for fetichism to be focused on inanimate objects, such as handkerchiefs, shoes, stockings, petticoats and hair ribbons, which are suggestive of the parts of the body upon which these objects are worn. There is a wide variation among people in the parts of the body upon which the attraction is centered.

The nature of the fetich is governed by unconscious memories that are formed very early in life. Normally these concealed memories lead one to admire certain features or characteristics of members of the opposite sex.

There are traces of fetichism, of varying degrees, in all human beings. When a man obtains satisfaction in saving the lock of hair, or glove or handkerchief of his sweetheart, or of someone else dear to him; and when a woman treasures the flower worn by her lover, we have examples of fetichism that are quite normal and socially acceptable. The mark of distinction between the abnormal and the normal, as in all other human characteristics, is one of degree rather than kind.

When an individual becomes obsessed so that his principal interest is concentrated on a certain part of the body that as no direct sexual significance, or more especially on a certain object, then it is recognized as the perverse condition, termed fetichism.

In its more pathological forms, the symbol has such a dominating influence over the fetich-worshipper that he prefers it to the part that it symbolizes. It is said that many fetichists, in order to indulge their fancies to the utmost, enter a business which gives them the maximum opportunity; thus some becoming shoe salesmen to realize their aim.

## *Exhibitionism*

In considering the exhibitionist component in our psychic make-up, we are interested only in its common manifestations. The pathological condition is when the subject secures conscious sexual gratification by displaying very personal parts of his anatomy. This form of perversion is not rare, and is the antithesis of the desire to see sexual objects—the abnormal type being designated as the *voyeur* or more popularly as "Peeping Tom."

It might be mentioned, incidentally, that in every individual there is a group of opposing traits that constitute the ego and sex properties of the individual, and the sum total of all these qualities constitute one's personality. These opposing traits, in the normal person, are so adjusted that they strike a satisfactory, workable equilibrium, so that the individual functions with as little friction as possible in his social relations. Conflicts, neurotic states, abnormalities and perversions, are a matter of maladjustment of some of these psychic components, the causes usually being deeply rooted in the experiences of early life.

Just to allude to a few of the factors involved, there are both heterosexual and homosexual tendencies (the latter being vestigial or rudimentary in the normal adult); there are qualities of exhibitionism and sexual curiosity; of sadism and masochism (the former in a degree is more peculiar to men and the latter to women) and others that are not so pronounced.

Examples of exhibitionism are so manifold and commonplace that we simply take them for granted without question. The manifestations are directed by the unconscious psychic processes and are a part of the secondary characteristics of sex. In this category, we recognize the propensity of women to wear low-necked dresses or gowns, short skirts, sleeveless waists, transparent fabrics, and similar dress effects, which permit more or less display of the flesh or figure, and thus afford an unconscious and frequently a conscious gratification of women's exhibitionist traits. Other examples of the same thing are elaborate hairdressing arrangements, picturesque hats, corsets (which were once supposed to emphasize the feminine shape), pointed shoes and high heels; various poses and attitudes, and other evidences that are considered to typify femininity.

Men also display exhibitionist qualities which are characteristic of their sex. Prominent among them are forms of dress which display or suggest masculine strength, such as square-cut or padded shoulders, athletic costumes and numerous actions and affectations which have as their motive the conscious and unconscious desire to attract the attention and win the admiration of the fair sex.

It is a conspicuous degree of exhibitionism in the ego-centre which spurs on certain persons of both sexes in their desire to take up acting, public speaking, lecturing, demonstrating or other callings of this general nature.

### Sadism and Masochism

Sadism (a term derived from Marquis de Sade, a French novelist who exploited perversions and cruelty of man to woman) is the psychic element which causes one to obtain satisfaction by inflicting pain on another. It is a positive force in our lives, and its operation is more manifold than we might like to acknowledge. It is expressed in the child who teases or injures cats, dogs and other pets, and, in a symbolical form, in destroying dolls and toy animals. It is an outstanding characteristic of the bully, and all individuals who subject others to acts of cruelty and punishment (even though it is "done for their own good"). In a lesser degree, it is manifested in tickling, teasing, and petty annoyances of a like nature. A very pronounced degree of sadism is shown by parents who whip their children;

men who beat their wives; boys who look for a
fight; successful soldiers, pugilists, football
players, and other physically aggressive persons.

In all its phases, sadism is probably the most
typical characteristic of the Caveman within us.
Undisguised, it is observed in the savage, who
glories in his cruelty, and exhibits the scalps he
has taken, or the skulls, as trophies worthy of
his valour. The "bad man" of the old frontier
who nicked the butt of his gun for every "man
that he got," is scarcely less pronounced in his
sadism. And their counterpart is with us today
in the gun-toting gangster of the modern city.
But we do not have to go to these criminal extremes to find positive sadistic traits. They are
present, actively and passively, in every individual, and it requires only the scratching of the
surface to reveal them undisguised.

In its purely sexual aspect, sadism is manifested by the individual. (usually male) who
obtains satisfaction by inflicting pain on his partner in the sex act. It may be evidenced in a very
slight degree, so that it gratifies the Unconscious
only or it may be more pronounced, causing real
pain or injury to the other party. The most extreme pathological form of sadism is typified in
the Jack-the-Ripper, who gratifies his perverted
passions by atrocious means, such as mutilating
or murdering his victim.

A perfect illustration of sadism, with the characteristic feelings of love and hate in operation,

is given in Oscar Wilde's version of *"Salomé."*
Having fallen madly in love with John, who spurns
her advances, she gratifies her craving by having
him beheaded. Then Salomé takes the severed
head and lavishes caresses upon it, as only the
degenerate sadist could.

Masochism (from L. von Sacher-Masoch, an
Austrian novelist, who described cruelty practised
on self) is also a characteristic inherent in every
one. While less noticeable in its manifestations
than sadism, its opposing trait, it is no less widespread. The two qualities are ever present in
every individual, although in widely varying proportions, and constitute one of the several ambivalent features which shape our personality.

There are individuals who are said to be glut-
tons for punishment. They can take beatings and
stand pain with great fortitude. In arduous
games and performances, such as football and
prize fights (already referred to under sadism)
the participants both give and take punishment
at the same time—and the ideal athlete is one
adept at both. In this way he shows his sadistic-
masochistic qualities. This is an expression of
the ego, rather than the sexual nature.

Masochism in its sexual phase is evidenced in
the person (usually female) who obtains sexual
gratification through being subjected to a certain
amount of pain during intercourse. The sex act
is usually accompanied by some slight suggestion
of pain to the woman, although in the proper

relations not the slightest harm or injury is done. However, there is a symbolic expression of this phenomenon—i.e. the mastery of the male and the submission of the female.

There are male masochists in the pervert class who experience sexual gratification by submitting to beatings—usually hiring prostitutes or others for that purpose.

Extreme cases of masochism and sadism have been laid to the witnessing by young children of their parents' embracing. Misunderstanding the nature of the act, the sometimes playful imitations of violence by the man and the suffering pretended by the woman may lead the child to commit in reality cruelty which the father only shammed, or another child to seek suffering which the mother seemed to feel. In short, the incident makes such an impression on the child that in his future sexual relations he unconsciously identifies himself with the apparently cruel father or the apparently abused mother.

When the natural sex instincts in mature adults are thwarted or suppressed, a substitute form of gratification is often obtained through masochistic-sadistic expressions. The early Christian ascetics, who denied themselves sexual intercourse, but found pleasure in flogging themselves (masochism) and others (sadism) offer a classic example of this abnormality. The same principle at work in a modified scale may be observed throughout history right down to the present. In the aggressive puritanical types and many ascetic reformers, we see persons whose morbid attitude toward natural phenomena, reacts in the form of petty persecutions and tyrannizing. Thus they find a really primitive outlet for an energetic force that is denied its normal expression.

The further the individual advances along cultural lines, the more his sadistic-masochistic characteristics may be sublimated into socially acceptable channels. A socially useful application of the sadistic tendencies is afforded in surgery, dentistry, the butcher business, and a variety of other callings. It is the masochistic trait which enables a normal person to render valuable service at the cost of pain or personal sacrifice, such as nursing or administering to the afflicted. Another and rarer example is in willingly going to jail or suffering punishment for a principle or to advance a cause.

### BIBLIOGRAPHY

LAY, WILFRID, *Man's Unconscious Passion*, New York, 1920.

BOUSFIELD, PAUL, *The Elements of Practical Psycho-Analysis*, New York, 1920.

FIELDING, WILLIAM J., *Sanity in Sex*, New York, 1920.

FREUD, SIGMUND, *Three Contributions to the Theory of Sex*, Nervous and Mental Disease Monograph No. 7.

SMITH, WM. HAWLEY, *Children by Chance or by Choice*, Boston, 1920.

TRIDON, ANDRÉ, *Psychoanalysis and Love*, New York, 1922.

# CHAPTER VIII

## THE CAVEMAN FRETTING

A wish earnestly desired,
Produced by will, and nourished
When gradually it must be thwarted
Burrows like an arrow in the flesh.
—GAUTAMA BUDDHA.

THERE is no end to the ills that have their origin in the Caveman's maladaptations. The progress of civilization has been possible only with the socialization of primitive, self-centered urges. Too often, however, these urges have not been socialized, or turned into some constructive outlet, but instead have been repressed.

The result of this commonplace tendency has been that the Caveman, denied a satisfactory means of expression, either primitive or social, has grown fretful and irritable under the restraint. The degree of minor afflictions ranges from mild irritability to chronic indisposition, depending upon the extent of the repressions.

These fretful ailments are usually designated as a manifestation of "nerves," and are considered to be the result of overwork, brain fag, fatigue, or rundown condition.

Accepting this popular diagnosis, it was natural

that the remedies prescribed should be "rest cures," tonics, experiments in dietetics and various innovations in short-cuts to health.

The inefficacy of these remedies is attested by the growing number of nervous cases in conjunction with the continued development of sanatoria, the everincreasing sale of "nerve-building" tonics and the popularity of dietetic and health fads.

## The Untiring Nerves

There is every reason to believe that the great mass of so-called "nervous disorders," including neurasthenia and other neurotic disturbances, is not the result of nerve exhaustion, brain exhaustion, or other form of mental strain or overwork.

According to the latest findings of the experimental psychologists and biologists, it does not appear that the brain and nerves can be exhausted by intellectual effort, *per se.*

In explanation of this apparently sweeping statement, to those who have experienced, or think they have experienced, brain fag from excessive mental effort, it may be added that mental exertion has no appreciable effect on the brain and the nerves, but instead reacts on the senses, the blood, the muscles and the flesh. Dr. Paul Du Bois, the eminent neurologist, has stated that among all his nervous cases, he has never found one which could be traced to intellectual overwork.

So far as the modern laboratory can discover, the nerves of the most confirmed neurotic are perfectly healthy. They are not injured, depleted or starved; the fatty sheath is unimpaired; there is no inflammation or accumulation of fatigue toxins, and the nerve cells are in every way intact.

The so-called "nervous diseases" are not symptoms of an unhealthy condition of the nerves, the brain, or spinal cord. On the other hand, they represent a state of misplaced, divided or uncontrollable interest and attention, and have their seat in the glands, the senses, the emotional mechanism, and the muscular tissues.

Where there is actual disintegration of the nerve structure, as in locomotor ataxia, the result is paralysis of the portion of the body controlled by the affected nerves. These afflictions comprise a very small percentage of human maladies; whereas the so-called "nervous disorders" outnumber all other ailments put together.

The nervous system seldom distinguishes between overwork and underwork. Neurasthenia is as apt to be associated with the latter as with the former. "Nervous disorders" in some instances may be *accompanied* by overwork, but they are not due to overwork, as we shall see. They are just as often found among people who have so little to do that killing time becomes monotonous.

The relationship between work and "nervous" troubles requires further elucidation. From the foregoing, it may be assumed that advice is given to those who are already working hard at some routine occupation, and think they are bordering on a nervous breakdown, to add a little bit more of the same kind of labor to their burden.

There is one essential requirement in making arduous work nerve-proof, and that is it must be interesting. This does not make it consume any less energy, but it means that work then becomes a source of satisfaction to the ego. As the ego is a factor of our primitive personality, we are again brought to the point where we must stress the necessity of coördinating the social and primitive sides of our personality. When the nature of our work is such that it accomplishes this result, there is no danger of nervous collapse from over-work.

Comparatively few people, however, are so fortunate as to have this kind of "job." With the rapid specialization of industry and business, the opportunities for expression of the personality and gratification of the ego at one's work are becoming more rare. The exceptions are to be found mostly in those fields that are devoted to experimentation and development, or that offer free play to the individual's initiative.

How can the person with the average routine job best obtain the ego gratification that is denied, or at best only partly satisfied, in working hours? If he feels his nerves on edge, and that he is over-worked, is it the part of wisdom to advise him to take the rest cure (if he can afford it) or get an easier job?

Barring those instances where the individual's work is obviously beyond his physical strength, and these are not "nervous" cases, it is not a question of overwork, and therefore "rest" is futile. The average person in this condition is suffering from maladaptation of his primitive nature—a lack of proper emotional outlet, combined with an attempt at self-coercion, which produces manifold complications in the personality.

A hobby that offers some *creative* possibilities, and that appeals to the particular bent of the individual, is undoubtedly the best "nerve bracer" to be found. If this is combined with an insight into the psychic and emotional processes, it will often affect a revolutionary change in disposition.

Not seldom a change of attitude, resulting in a more ready adaptability to the inevitable, is realized in a personal crisis. This accounts for the beneficial results obtained so frequently from Christian Science, New Thought, and other cults which operate through suggestion. The emotional appeal is so often responded to at some period in the individual's life when the emotional nature is at its height, as at a climacteric or during an illness. Consequently, a part of the personality that had been denied an adequate outlet is now vouchsafed a means of expression, with untold benefit to the organism as a whole.

Many people with a more strictly rational turn of mind (as contrasted with the emotional), who obtain a real insight into their psychic operations, secure similar advantages by turning their released energy into channels of scientific interest.

## *The Œdipus Complex*

The Œdipus, of all the complexes, has been found to be the link which most frequently binds the individual to the past, drawing him back to an infantile goal of satisfaction. This archaic desire in the soul of the male, Freud has named in recognition of its analogy to the tragedy of King Œdipus, who, according to Sophocles, by fate killed his father and won his mother for a wife. It has its female counterpart in the Electra complex. Electra, according to Euripides, took revenge on her mother for the murder of the husband because she was in this way deprived of her father.

As the psychological reaction is the same in each instance, the term Œdipus complex is often used interchangeably for both situations, it being understood that the sex of the parent is the opposite to that of the child.

Leaving aside the more severe pathological cases, there are still to be found in the general run of neurotic afflictions a countless host of people who are influenced by this nuclear or root complex, so called because its influence is so powerful that it seems a determining factor in facing many of the problems of life.

Biography offers an interesting study of many famous characters who were influenced profoundly by the Œdipus complex. Some of these instances may be observed in Chapter XV, in connection with neurotic and pathological tendencies in men of genius. The older writers and biographers themselves did not realize the underlying psychological motive, and that makes it the more interesting to read the unrecognized "complexes" interpreted so accurately from the facts at hand.

Just one illuminating example will suffice. We are told that one of Pascal's idiosyncrasies was that he could not bear to see his father and mother together; they had to approach him separately. We see here the unconscious jealousy toward his father and the desire to be the sole love of his mother. The complex was so powerful that the association of ideas brought about by the presence of both parents produced an unbearable conflict. By seeing his parents separately, the love-jealousy (Œdipus) complex was not so strongly moved.

### Worry and Fear

Worry is the outstanding characteristic of the neurotic, and worry is merely another name for fear. The most groundless fears are seized upon by the neurotic mind, and translated into mountains of worry. If there is positively nothing real or tangible to worry about, then the imagination will quickly overcome the deficiency. No better example of this has been instanced than that given by Dostoevsky, the Russian novelist: "There was a frightful fear of something which I cannot define, of something which I cannot conceive, which does not exist, but which rises before me as a horrible, distorted, inexorable and irrefutable fact."

Invariably it will be found that there is some hidden complex responsible for these groundless fears. When a person is "touchy" about something, it is evidence that there is a complex connected with it. The ideas around which have gathered the painful emotions are buried deep in the Unconscious. Ordinarily, they escape into consciousness only occasionally, and are identified by their sensitiveness regarding some particular subject.

The variety of obsessional fears is infinite, but there are certain kinds so typical that they have been classified. Among these symptoms of psychoneurosis, sometimes referred to as psychasthenia, are agoraphobia, fear of open spaces; claustrophobia, fear of closed spaces; astrapaphobia, fear of thunder and lightning; aerophobia, fear of being in high places; erythrophobia, fear of red (indicating selfreproach, or shame of some kind); morbid desires for drink or drugs; pyromania, impulse to set fire to things; arithmomania, impulse to count everything; onomatomania, impulse to repeat one word, and so on.

Dr. Morton Prince (*The Unconscious*) described the case of a lady who had an intense fear of white cats. Characteristically, the lady could not account for the fear. It was finally traced, however, to an incident which happened thirty-five years before, when, at the age of five or six she was very much frightened by a white kitten which had a fit while she was playing with it.

A reproach for some act done in childhood, if severly repressed, may develop into an anxiety neurosis, with hypochondriacal tendencies, and a consciousness of shame, which may color one's whole outlook on life. This suggests the desirability of attempting to reason with children when they transgress, thereby giving them a rational basis for their conduct, instead of censuring without consideration for the child's feelings.

The old-fashioned religious training which involved threats of eternal damnation and all sorts of dire punishment for doing this and that, or for not doing so and so, must have been the cause of unnumbered psychic disturbances built up on repressions and phobias. It was generally ineffective, inasmuch as it apparently did not lessen infractions of the ethical code, and at the same time it established a law of personal conduct based on fear—with all its evil concomitants—instead of intelligent understanding.

In *Varieties of Religious Experience*, William James quotes Emerson as saying: "Our young people are diseased with the theological problems of original sin, origin of evil, predestination, and the like. These never presented a practical difficulty to any man, never darkened across any man's road, who did not go out of his way to seek them. They are the soul's mumps and measles and whooping-cough.''

There has been during the past few decades a pronounced let-up in the old attitude of frightening people into an alleged godliness, although, taking the world at large, there are still in effect too many remnants of this sinister policy.

The ghosts of ancient fears are still rampant. The phantoms of needless worry still haunt untold numbers of people. Who will not recognize the universal application of the following expressive thought from Goethe (*Faust*)?

As water, fire, as poison, steel,
We dread the blows we never feel,
And what we never lose is yet by us lamented!

### Neurotic Negativism

Because the average neurotic is obsessed by indefinite, and sometimes indefinable, fears and cravings; because he is unable to adapt himself to the demands of reality, he becomes a ready victim to negativism. The most common aspect of negativism is in stressing, usually in an exaggerated manner, the mistakes and faults of others. In fact, it is typical of the neurotic to project his own shortcomings upon other persons, i.e., he criticises them for failings of which he himself is guilty. There is a keen bit of insight evidenced in the wise old maxim, "negation is a sign of the small mind."

Petty disparagement is among the most common of the popular vices, while ancient wrongs may continue unmolested. The reason for this is that the latter is sanctified by precedent, and precedent is the sacred cow of negativism.

It is no empty pastime that the neurotic indulges in when he belittles the efforts of those about him. It is a source of substitute gratification to his ego urge, which lacks the energetic consistency to achieve a positive form of gratification by creative effort. This "sour grapes" attitude, or the tendency to pour cold water on the accomplishments of others, enhances the neurotic critic's estimation of himself. Instead of achieving superiority by socially useful acts and deeds, he gains a spurious form of superiority by lowering the prestige of those about him. By pulling others down, he fancies himself raised to a higher plane.

Nietzsche, in *Human, All Too Human,* has appraised this form of disparagement in the following words: "In order to maintain their self-respect in their own eyes and a certain thoroughness of action, not a few men, perhaps the majority, find it absolutely necessary to run down and disparage all their acquaintances."

We are all familiar with the individual who

greets every new idea and innovation with scorn. He prides himself upon his perspicacity and shrewdness—he "has to be shown"—whereas, he is merely the embodiment of futile pessimism. He is negation personified. His satisfaction is secured in passing judgment upon the ideas of the day. He promptly condemns them, and by so dóing proves (to himself) his own superiority over those who have gained public notice.

Negativism is a phase of the neurotic's struggle with reality. Indeed, it is often an attempt at expression of his personality, but it is a vain attempt. So much of his energy is consumed in internal conflicts that there is no possibility while these conflicts last for a positive application, or a constructive outlet, of his vital urges. The primitive side of the personality is fretting under the leaden inhibitions and repressions. Community interests and the ethical code of the individual do not permit the Caveman to express himself in his aboriginal fashion, and the lack of adaptation to social requirements prevents the alternative of a socially acceptable mode of expression.

BIBLIOGRAPHY

JACKSON, JOSEPHINE A. and HELEN M. SALISBURY, *Outwitting Our Nerves*, New York, 1921.
CORIAT, I., *Repressed Emotions*, New York, 1920.
WHITE, WILLIAM A., *Principles of Mental Hygiene*, New York, 1916.

WHITE, WILLIAM A., *Elements of Character Formation,*
New York.

FIELDING, WILLIAM J., *The Puzzle of Personality,*
Girard, Kansas, 1922.

PIERCE, FREDERICK, *Our Unconscious Mind and How to
Use It.* New York, 1922.

# CHAPTER IX

## THE CAVEMAN SICK

*Hamlet to Laertes—*
  Was't Hamlet wrong'd Laertes? Never Hamlet:
  If Hamlet from himself be ta'en away,
  And when he's not himself does wrong Laertes,
  Then Hamlet does it not; Hamlet denies it.
  Who does it then? His madness: if 't be so,
  Hamlet is of the faction that is wrong'd;
  His madness is poor Hamlet's enemy.
                          —SHAKESPEARE.

THE Caveman sick has long baffled the sciences of therapeutics and the arts of healing. The difficulty has been primarily in the failure to understand and account for the duality of human nature. Symptoms have been diagnosed almost exclusively from the standpoint of conscious ideas and ideals, from a superficial observation of the functions of the vital organs, and without any adequate conception of the basic unconscious forces upon these organs.

As a result, myriads of patients have been treated for functional disturbances, and even organic diseases, when the trouble has been in psychic maladjustments of the most elemental character, rather than with the physical organism. Of course, these disorders emanating from the unconscious psychic processes are reflected in pronounced physical symptoms, which in turn are in themselves distressing. They become, in fact, the recognized seat of far-reaching disabilities, and practically all attention has been given to this apparent causation, while the real cause remained hidden.

Some of the lesser effects of unconscious conflicts and repressions have been alluded to in the preceding chapter. Every individual experiences these in a degree, as there is always a certain amount of conflict between the primitive biological urges and the demands of organized society (and one's ethical concepts). Normally, however, there is the possibility of a satisfactory adjustment and adaptation, insuring a well-balanced personality and a healthy, useful life.

### The Libido

It is when the vital, energetic factor of the organism, which Freud terms the *libido,* becomes blocked, that a conflict ensues. This dynamic life-force must have an outlet, or it will play havoc with the psychic processes, with the resultant physical symptoms already referred to.

Dr. Eduard Hitschmann has remarked that a dammed-up libido hunts out a weak place and breaks through, expressing itself in neurotic substitute gratification. The point to remember is that it *will express itself,* if the subject is at all vital, so it would seem to be the rational thing to direct it into some useful, socially acceptable course. The alternatives are outlets through vicious, anti-social channels, or neurotic "substitute gratification", that is destructive to the personality and a trial to those with whom the victim comes in contact.

The ceaseless flow of impulses or discharge of psychic energy which animates the human organism, becomes involved in conflicts through the mechanism known as the pleasure principle and the reality principle.

According to the first principle, we instinctively accept the pleasurable and reject the painful, without regard to the ultimate results. This is the expression of the Caveman in his pristine glory. In any organized society, in fact in any group-life, a complete acceptance of the pleasure principle would result in the individual's quick destruction (unless cared for as an infant, or confined as an adult), because he would be in constant conflict with his environment. This principle in its true sense eliminates all consideration for others, hence it is anti-social, egotistical. In a modified form, of course, i.e., in a socially acceptable manner, it is necessary for every individual to express his primitive personality more often than we may imagine.

The reality principle demands that we accept some painful experiences, because in so doing we adjust ourselves to the requirements of social life.

It involves consideration for the rights of others. It is the mainspring of altruistic and idealistic actions—the highest expressions of the cultural personality.

The pleasure principle has its biological foundation in the life-urge of the individual. It is *individualistic*. It represents the primary, original form of mental activity. It is innate and spontaneous in its manifestations, and is characteristic of the earliest stages of human development, both in the individual and the race. It is typically expressed in the mental life of the infant, and to a less extent in the savage. In the infant, nothing but its own desires concern it, and it demands with unqualified insistence their fulfilment in the shape of food, warmth, petty attentions and any object it may notice.

The reality principle is the expression of the welfare and continuity of the group. It is *social*. If the individual were not capable of acting upon the reality principle to a very large degree throughout life, he would as a consequence cease to exist.

Man must realize the uncompromising force of sea, air, fire, gravity, wild animals, in order to maintain life. He must recognize the claims, needs and, superior force of his fellow-men, even in the most primitive society or community.

Thus in every act of living, even without thinking about it, we are gathering consciously and unconsciously a working knowledge of the reality principle. It is exemplified in the old adage of "learning by experience."

It is the inevitable conflict between these two principles in our psychic stream that is the cause of repressions. And repressions which become so severe that they cause serious disharmony in the Unconscious result in hysteria, neuroses, psychoses, insanity. This is another way of saying that, because he has been deprived of adequate expression, the Caveman is sick.

Society has shut off the opportunity for the functioning of the primitive personality in its original form; and the neurotic individual's irrational training has made difficult or impossible a form of expression that is socially acceptable. So the Old Adam breaks out in the disguise of aggravating physical symptoms or mental aberrations.

### Physical Symptoms of Neuroses

Only a few of the physical disabilities that may be simulated by psychoneuroses, as a result of intense repressions of natural urges, are heart disorders, headache, rapid respiration, hay fever, constipation, diarrhœa, indigestion, nausea, vomiting, insomnia, diabetes, menstrual troubles, impotence, backache, asthma, sore throat, abnormal motor activities, blushing, not to mention many less common.

Some very unusual physical symptoms also

have been definitely traced to hysterical sources. There is the case of a woman patient who was apparently suffering from a tumor. The swelling was present in a most pronounced form, and the pain severe. An operation was decided upon, and on administering the ether, the swelling vanished. The "tumor" had disappeared. It was an hysterical "growth." It is probable that some sensitive complex was touched on a certain occasion when she had read or heard of a tumor, with the result that the idea obsessed her, and her Unconscious responded to her fears by counterfeiting a "tumor."

Morbid experiences of early childhood, or infancy, often contribute to the most puzzling cases of neuroses in adulthood. The incident has been repressed out of consciousness because of its unpleasant nature. The impressions it has created, however, remain active below the level of consciousness, and the resultant festering psychic discharge is accompanied by various pathological symptoms.

Pfister mentions the case of a girl sixteen years old who suffered regularly at her menstrual periods from vomiting. It was found that when a child she had gained the impression that children are born through the mouth. After enlightenment in this particular, the symptom immediately ceased and did not reappear.

Instances of phantom pregnancy have been known where the patient manifested all the symptoms of the parturient condition, even in an advanced stage. This, like countless other forms of hysteria, is due to obsessive thoughts on the subject until the expectation becomes fulfilled in a symbolical way.

## Disturbance of Sexual Processes

The neuroses have been divided into the true neuroses and the psycho-neuroses.

The true neuroses are neurasthenia and anxiety neuroses. According to Freud, these diseases are caused by a disturbance of the sexual processes, which determine the formation and utilization of the sexual libido.

He summarizes the situation in the following words: "We can hardly avoid perceiving these processes as being, in their last analysis, chemical in their nature, so that we recognize in the true neuroses the somatic effect of disturbances in the sexual metabolism, while in the psycho-neuroses, we recognize besides the psychic effects of the same disturbances. The resemblance of the neuroses to the manifestations of intoxication and abstinence, following certain alkaloids, and to Basedow's and Addison's diseases obtrudes itself clinically without any further ado, and just as these two diseases should no longer be described as nervous diseases, so will the genuine neuroses soon have to be removed from this class, despite their nomenclature."

In the opinion of Freud, neurasthenia is due to exaggerated sexual self-gratification which weakens the individual's will-power by making the goal too easily obtainable, affords inadequate relief, diminishes potency and, by ignoring too many psychological sources of excitement, may cause physical injury. The victim thus becomes anti-social and betrays the result of his vain strife against passion in many ways, lack of will power, doubts about the possibility of achievement and self-reproaches.

The usual symptoms of anxiety neurosis are general irritability, exaggerated visual and auditory sensations which are frequently the cause of sleeplessness, anxious expectations of accidents, death, insanity, accompanied in some cases by a disturbance of one or more bodily functions, respiration, circulation, glandular functions, and so on. Dizziness, which never quite leads to complete loss of equilibrium, is one of the most characteristic symptoms of anxiety neurosis.

The relation between the general lack of rational sex enlightenment and the wide prevalence of neurotic disturbances is seen when we consider Freud's contention that the symptoms of anxiety neurosis are substitutes for the specific action which follows natural sexual excitement and which is accompanied by acceleration of respiration, palpitation, sweating and congestion.

Thus it is found that men who resort to ungratifying forms of sexual activity, and women left unsatisfied by the impotence or *ejaculatio præcox* of their husbands, are often sufferers from anxiety neurosis.

Sometimes this result will not become manifest for years in people who have unsatisfactory sexual relations. However, when they are confronted with a critical situation or are forced to undergo a trying ordeal, an anxiety neurosis suddenly settles upon them. For years, they have been preparing the ground-work for this condition, and it requires only the stimulus of a troublesome experience to start off the mechanism of a pronounced neurosis.

Anxiety neurosis, too, is commonly attributed to over-work. This phase of the question has been touched upon in the preceding chapter. Freud again offers a suggestion pertinent in this domain when he states that the physician who informs a busy man that he has overworked himself, or an active woman that her household duties have been too burdensome, should tell his patients they are sick, not because they have sought to discharge duties which for a civilized brain are comparatively easy, but because they have neglected, if not stifled, their sexual life while attending to their duties.

The psycho-neuroses are hysteria and obsessions. They are repeatedly traced back to erotic experiences in childhood; hence, to the influence of unconscious or repressed idea-complexes.

Hysteria is more psychic, and neurasthenia more toxic—but both have a sexual basis.

Anxiety hysteria is frequently associated with hysteria proper. In this case, the anxiety arises not only from physical sources, but from a part of the ungratified desire which embraces a number of the complexes.

As the normal mind reacts to danger through anxiety, it may be considered analogous that in this case the mind is defending itself against fancied internal danger. The psychic mechanism is the same as in hysteria, except that it does not lead to conversion into physical symptoms. Anxiety hysteria invariably tends to develop a phobia.

The obsessional neurosis is featured by constant ambivalence, or the experiencing of opposite feelings at the same time, such as love and hatred for the same person, although one of these emotions may dominate in the Conscious and the other in the Unconscious.

Hysteria is more peculiar to the female sex, and obsessional neurosis to the male sex.

### The Psychoses

In the psychoses, we find widely varying degrees of insanity, whereas in the neuroses we may observe every conceivable degree of mental variation from almost normal rationality down to the borderland of irresponsibility, with frequent lapses over the brink.

Dr. Alfred Adler emphasizes the difference between the neuroses and psychoses in the following words: "Longing for an unattainable ideal is at the bottom of both. Defeat or fear of defeat causes the weaker individual to seek a substitute for his real goal. At this point begins the process of psychic transformation designated as a neurosis. In the neurosis, the pursuit of the fictitious goal does not lead to an open conflict with reality, the neurotic simply considering reality as a very disturbing element, as he does in neurasthenia, hypochondria, anxiety, compulsion neurosis and hysteria. In the psychoses, the guiding masculine fiction appears disguised in pictures and symbols of infantile origin. The patient no longer acts as though he wished to be masculine, to be above, but as though he had already attained those ends."

In short, the neurotic is grieved by not being all-powerful. The psychotic *is* all-powerful, and attempts to force his environment to share his belief.

In order to obtain a true conception of the psychoses (insanity)—which condition is most literally the Caveman sick—it is necessary to compare them with certain attitudes of the Caveman in the "normal" individual. In the insane patient, we find a prolonged or permanent dissociation in which the primitive personality is in the ascendency. Normally the primitive personality asserts itself *unmasked* in dreams, and in a number of more restricted ways that have been described.

We find that the mind of the insane patient functions in his waking hours in a manner quite identical with the *mind of the sane person in his sleep.*

In our dreams we are temporarily irrational, illogical, supremely egotistical and self-centered. These characteristics are constant with the insane (or intermittent in cases where the victim is subject to insane attacks with lucid intervals).

Kant remarked that "the lunatic is a dreamer in the waking state." The same thought was expressed by A. Krauss, the psychiatrist, in slightly different language, namely: "Insanity is a dream with the senses awake."

We are told by Wundt, the noted psychologist, that "as a matter of fact, we may in the dream ourselves live through almost all the symptoms which we meet in the insane asylum." Schopenhauer termed the dream a short insanity, and insanity a long dream.

In convalescence from insanity, it has been observed that while the functions of the day are normal, the dream life may belong to the psychoses.

Another characteristic of insanity is the tendency toward infantile regression. This is also typical, to a lesser extent, in the neurotic. In fact, insanity, except when due to disintegration of the brain structure (such as may result from syphilitic lesion, alcoholic deterioration, tumor or other malignant growth) is essentially an extreme neurotic condition.  It has all the symptoms, in an exaggerated form, of the various neuroses. It is almost invariably the neurotic, barring the cases due to physiological causes as indicated above, who become insane as they gradually lose their grip on the vitals of reality.

### Graduations of Insanity

We are again impressed with the fact that there is no hard and fast dividing line between the sane and the insane.  Even people considered highly rational have fits of rage that evidence all the features of insanity while they last.  Individuals with pretty good practical minds sometimes do some very irrational or foolish things when seized by an unaccountable impulse—even to the extent of committing murder or suicide, as has been known to happen.

It is understood, of course, that we are discussing acquired insanity, known as *dementia,* as congenital mental defectiveness (*idiocy, imbecility,* etc.) is altogether outside of the scope of this work.

As a general rule, the more thoroughly insane the person is, the more infantile he becomes in his actions.  Cases are not uncommon where the victim regresses so far, and becomes so detached from all interest in life that he lies down, utterly disregarding his environment and all the bodily functions, even assuming perhaps the prenatal position of the fetus.

The biological aspect of the regression to insanity is also apparent. If the prehistoric troglodyte could be transported to our midst, his every act would in our eyes brand him as insane. He would be absolutely out of harmony with his twentieth century environment, and in all probability completely unadaptable. In the paleolithic age, he may have been a useful member of his primitive community, but in the maze of a highly intricate society, he would be as useless as the most hopeless inmate of a modern Bedlam.

In other chapters, we have reviewed some of the ineradicable biological memories which lie dormant under our cultural veneer, and which are revived when the conditions are favorable. What is more plausible than that the human organism (considering it as a physical and psychic entity), when the faculty of rational discretion is removed, should revert to the uncensored mode of conduct of ages past? Mankind's ancient biological heritage is then revived in its primordial form with the loss of the rationally developed faculties.

It is always an unbearable emotional shock, or series of shocks, which produces the trauma or psychic wound resulting in insanity. There is invariably present, of course, the neurotic predisposition which causes the subject to fall so readily a victim. The more adaptable person adjusts himself to situations which produce a profound psychic shock in the neurotic. The mechanism is usually repression, and symbolization (a powerful factor in the unconscious) plays an important part in the patient's irrational expressions.

Practically all types and degrees of insanity afford proof of some repression at work, although the conflict is often so deeply buried that the primary cause may not be found. The symbolization, the outward manifestation of the psychosis, however, frequently gives a clue.

Dr. C. G. Jung, the Zurich analytic psychologist, has instanced a case in which his patient manifested a high degree of symbolization of the "stereotyped action" order. An old woman, who had been an inmate of the institution for many years, occupied her whole waking time in a single stereotyped performance. She was never heard to speak, nor had she shown the slightest interest in anything that occurred around her. She sat all day long in a huddled position, continuously moving her arms and hands in a manner suggestive of a shoemaker engaged in sewing shoes. All her waking hours were absorbed in these movements which were repeated with unvarying regularity and monotony from one year's end to another.

When the woman's history was investigated it was found that as a young girl she had been engaged to be married, and that the engagement was suddenly broken off. The great emotional shock resulting from this occurrence completely unbalanced her mind, and she remained in this state of insanity during the remainder of her life. It was further learned that her faithless lover had been a shoemaker by trade.

It has been said that *ideas* are the most potent forces with which mankind deals. Constructive ideas, carried into effect, are responsible for every bit of the world's progress. But, on the other hand, false, destructive ideas, or negative ideas, have been responsible for the greater part of the misery that has afflicted man. And it is the false, irrational ideas that have been inculcated in the minds of the young, and kept on being hammered into the minds of the matured, that are responsible for the ills in the psychic domain, no less than in the physical world.

Most neuroses and psychoses are diseased ideas (or false ideas which have created a diseased state of mind) that have been absorbed in the experience of the individual. Chiefly they have been kicked in by organized society. And with a sort of fatalistic retribution, they in time turn upon society and wreak their vengeance.

Man has remained in ignorance of natural laws, particularly those relating to his instinctive modes of action, and he has paid the price. He has ignored and abused, or attempted to suppress, the elemental part of himself, his primitive personality, with the result that the Caveman within has thrown on the organism the burden of a sick and disordered patient.

### BIBLIOGRAPHY

FREUD, SIGMUND, *Selected Papers on Hysteria and Other Psychoneuroses*, Nervous and Mental Disease Monograph Series No. 4.

HITSCHMANN, EDUARD, *Freud's Theory of the Neuroses*, New York, 1917.

WHITE, WILLIAM A., *Outlines of Psychiatry*, Nervous and Mental Disease Monograph Series No. 1.

JELLIFFE, SMITH ELY, *Technique of Psychoanalysis*, Nervous and Mental Disease Monograph Series No. 26.

# CHAPTER X

# THE CAVEMAN'S RELIGIOUS HERITAGE

Heaven's but the Vision of fulfilled Desire,
And Hell the Shadow from a Soul on fire
Cast on the Darkness into which ourselves
So late emerg'd from, shall so soon expire.
—OMAR KHAYYAM, *The Rubaiyat.*

RELIGIOUS traditions are undoubtedly the oldest of all existing traditions. The recognized essentials of religion have changed little because the primitive personality of man has changed little. And it is the primitive personality, the emotional side of human nature, that is religious in the commonly accepted sense of the word.

The emotions are essentially static, expressing themselves normally along the stereotyped grooves of biological habit and social tradition. On the other hand, it is the intellect (the cultural personality) that is dynamic, progressive. The conflict between intellectual progress and theology, i.e., organized religion, is proverbial. The older and more orthodox churches tacitly admit this conflict—although they may deny impeding scientific progress—by cherishing their ancient dogma, even to the extent, as some of them do, of claiming they "never change."

189

The oldest form of religious expression we know of is Nature worship in its many phases. It is probable that the first gleaming of intelligence stood in awe before the mysteries of nature, and crudely speculated as to the source of life.

There seems to be nothing visible or imaginable that man has not worshipped at some period. He has sanctified an infinite variety of objects of nature, including animals and fishes, trees and stones, flowers and fruits, the sun, moon, planets and the stars, and Man himself. There are still savage tribes in remote parts of the earth who follow some variation of this primordial practice.

### Phallic Worship

Among the earliest known forms of religious worship is Phallicism, in which the generative organs are adored. There are still in existence remarkable specimens of original phallic symbols, and the extent which this symbolization has been woven into the arts and architecture, and the literature, languages and traditions of the race, is beyond reckoning. A great amount of data on this subject has been collected by Dr. Lee Alexander Stone, an eminent American authority on phallic lore to whom I am indebted for numerous helpful suggestions in the preparation of the material in this chapter.

Within the period of early civilization, Phallicism was practiced by the Egyptians, Phœnicians, Pompeians and Greeks. Phallic images are found among the ruins of these ancient races. This form of nature worship had its variation in the belief in the fertilizing effect of the sun and rain upon the earth, and in the association of human sexual interests with the fertility of fields. The rites connected with the worship of Baal and Ashtaroth (gods mentioned in the Bible) had their basis in the belief that growth of vegetation was favourably influenced by sexual practices.

The cross, one of the most venerated of all religious symbols, is to be found on ancient monuments throughout Egypt and India, as well as in other parts of the world. Before white men set foot upon the Western Hemisphere, tribes of both North and South American Indians used the cross as a symbol in their worship.

Phallic symbols have been found in widely scattered parts of the American continent; large stone phalli having been dug up in Tennessee, Georgia, California, and other places in the United States, British Columbia and Mexico. Many of these specimens are in the National Museum at Washington.

Talismans and amulets carved in the image of the phallus were common in the ancient world. It was customary among the higher classes to carve them out of precious metals and gem stones in exact likeness of the organs they symbolized. The wearing of these symbols was believed to add to the virility of the wearer, and to ward off danger. The survival of this belief (at least an unconscious belief, when not conscious) is evidenced in the continued popularity of charms, talismans and amulets down to the present day.

### Phallic Symbolism in Architecture

General J. G. R. Forlong, in his *Rivers of Life,* refers to two mounds in Kentucky that are undoubtedly of phallic origin, and compares them with phallic mounds in Egypt. The pyramids and obelisks of the latter country are also known to be phallic representations.

There are many phallic symbols perpetuated in the finest architecture, and it is significant, in consideration of our present subject, that nowhere are they found in more profusion than in modern, as well as ancient, churches and cathedrals. The steeple and spire are distinctly phallic in origin, so that in these essentials to the modern church, we find preserved symbols of nature worship that long preceded Christianity or any other existing religion.

There is a conventional design of doors and windows and ornamental apertures in churches that is an almost faithful duplication of the primitive symbols of the external female genitals. The extent that other phallic symbolization is expressed in minor details of church ornamentation quite beggars description.

Among the richest fields of phallic symbolism

to be found today are the cemeteries. As the religious influence is paramount in cemetery monumental decorations, we are once more brought face to face with the survival of the most ancient of symbols. Modern man has solved many of the mysteries of nature, but on the question of the first cause of life, and in facing the ultimate physical reaction of death, he stands in practically the same helpless position as did his prehistoric ancestor. And, instinctively, unconsciously, he has acted similarly to his early progenitors. The monuments and shafts and crosses and conventional ornamentation of the cemetery, with their unbroken traditions from early antiquity, are the mute expression of his wonder over the riddle of creation and of his hope for immortality.

The use of the horseshoe as a symbol of protection against "bad luck" had its origin in the ancient custom of using the figure of the female organ to ward off evil influences. Even down to the Middle Ages in Western Europe, it was the custom to nail this symbol over the entrance to buildings as a protection against the dreaded evil eye and witchcraft.

Among the Arabs of Northern Africa, it was a common practice to place over the door of the house or tent the generative organ of a mare, cow or female camel as a protecting talisman. As the figure of this member is more susceptible to mutilation in form than that of the male, especially in the crude workmanship of untrained handymen, it gradually assumed shapes quite far removed from the original model, but nevertheless true in its symbolization.

It is plain that the figure of the female organ readily lent itself to the rude form of a horseshoe, and in time was substituted by the real horseshoe, which we so often find nailed over doors. Certain triangles, triple loops and other similar decorative devices and architectural ornaments are doubtless variations of the same primitive object.

### *Universality of Symbols*

Primitive man and early civilized man formulated their ideas in symbolical pictures, and to this day symbols are the natural language of our primitive personality. In the chapter on dreams, the significance of symbolism has been mentioned.

The erotic expressions of the ancients were so little disguised that the sexual aspect of their symbols is almost always obvious. It can be perceived in their myths, legends and folk-stories. Today, the basic motive of surviving symbols is more concealed, although the sexual phase will invariably be found with a little scrutiny.

To recur to dream representation, in the phantasies of our sleep, the human body is often indicated by a building, house or church. The male body is represented by flat surfaces, smooth walls over which one may climb, and the female body by set tables, walls with balconies, mounds, hills, a rolling landscape.

The male genitals may be symbolized by various elongated objects, sticks, tree-trunks, pillars, towers, steeples, fruits or vegetables of like shape, and birds, fishes, snakes and all sharp weapons. The female genitals are represented by shoes, boxes, caves, stoves, windows, doors, closets and gardens.

Poetry and art which call, to so great an extent, upon the resources of the unconscious mind, furnish excellent examples of symbolization that rival some of the phantastic dreams of our sleep.[1] The following lines from a poem, *I Have Been Through The Gates,* by Charlotte Mew (Macmillan Co., 1921), offer a perfect illustration of pure symbolization, with the sexual significance strikingly in evidence:

> His heart, to me was a place of places and
>   pinnacles and shining towers;
> I saw it then as we see things in dreams—I
>   do not remember how long I slept;
> I remember the trees, and the high, white
>   walls, and how the sun was always on the
>   towers;
> The walls are standing today, and the gates;
>   I have been through the gates; I have
>   groped, I have crept
> Back, back. . . .

[1] See Mörike's poem *The Maiden's First Love Song,* page 89, Chapter IV.

Life today, no less than in the past, is made brighter for the Caveman by examples of symbolization that we scarcely recognize as such. These acts satisfy our unconscious desires for primitive expression, often without the least conscious inkling of their real underlying significance. For instance, we throw rice and old shoes at newlyweds without comprehending the true meaning of the act. Consciously we are following an established custom, but unconsciously we are doing something more important. We are giving expression in a symbolical way to a wish that is quite appropriate for the occasion, and which our conventional ethics would not permit us to express in a more direct way.

During all ages and in the folklore of all races, shoes have been a symbol of the female genitals, and rice (or wheat or other common cereal) the symbol of the male fructifying seed. Hence, we unconsciously indicate the sexual character of the new relationship with the normal outcome of fruitfulness or prolificacy, which the conventions of modern society would not permit us openly to mention.

### Symbolism in Ceremonies

Many existing formalities in connection with marriage are acts of symbolism descended from remote antiquity. The wedding ring is a symbol of what once was the yoke of man's absolute authority over the newly acquired spouse. The orange blossoms—significantly from one of the most prolific of all fruit-bearing trees—is plainly a symbol meant to bring fruitfulness to the union. The father or other male member of the family usually "gives the bride away," which is reminiscent of the time when woman had literally no say in the matter. The honeymoon tour, beginning with the hasty departure after the ceremony, symbolizes the act of carrying the bride away—which was once a procedure involving the use of strategy, force and flight.

There is also a symbolic significance in the betrothal, and a high degree of it in the rites of baptism, and even more in the ceremonies and obsequies performed over the dead.

### Symbolism in Numbers

Certain numbers have exercised a profound influence over the human mind, without regard to time or race, as also have certain characterizations. These have been emphasized in religions, and their real origin is in their mystical attraction to the primitive mind. The number "three" is notable. There is the Holy Trinity; the Three Wise Men; Jesus, Mary and Joseph; Christ and the two thieves; Faith, Hope and Charity. The Crucifixion took place at three o'clock; the Resurrection occurred on the third day; Peter denied

Christ three times; Peter had a vision thrice repeated (Acts x).

The note of importance or of finality which this number carries leads to its constant emphasis in daily life. Only to mention a few instances, we have "the third and last warning", "ready, set, go", "ready, aim, fire", "three strikes and out", and a drowning person "comes up three times", the proverbial cat has "nine lives" (three times three), etc.

At a very early period, man was believed to be a trinity, made up of "body, soul and spirit." The "salt, sulphur and mercury" of the ancient alchemists undoubtedly referred to man as being composed of a trinity of elements. And this central concept has been projected upon the Divinity. In this connection, Schelling says: "The philosophy of mythology proves that a trinity of divine potentialities is the root from which have grown the religious ideas of all nations of any importance that are known to us."

Another number that always has had a special significance is "seven." In *Revelation,* we find mention of seven candlesticks, a book with seven seals, seven stars, seven angels with seven horns, a dragon with seven heads, seven vials, and seven plagues; and John addressed a document to the seven churches of Asia.

In everyday life, we speak of the seven seas, the seven wonders of the world. Salome wore seven veils, the week has seven days, people reach their majority at three times seven years, and the allotted age of man is seven decades.

Abstract ideas and institutions are given personal names symbolic of the parent image. The Church is the "Mother," also the "Bride." There are the "Heavenly Father" and the "Holy Mother." These are analogous, in nationalistic characterization, to such terms as "Mother Country", "Fatherland", "Uncle Sam."

## Symbols—Language of Primitive Personality

It is very likely that the Church fathers, in adopting ancient rites to their ceremonies, acted largely from unconscious motives rather than from conscious imitation. Symbolization is the language that is universally understood by the primitive personality. The human race has always clung to established traditions, and when one system of society has succeeded another, it has invariably utilized much of the formality of the preceding order, even though there may have been a radical change in principle. So it is that religious institutions, following the course of all organic social life, have built their structure around the emotional life of the people, utilizing those traditions that had become intrenched in the primitive mind.

There is no other social agency that offers mankind so free an outlet for a symbolical expression of his primitive nature as religion. Not only are the architectural features, in a symbolical form, associated with humanity's earliest devotions, but the whole atmosphere of ecclesiasticism is steeped in the Past. The sacred books cover a period of history when the social organization was comparatively simple, man's mode of life elemental, and his abstract thoughts were expressed in mythological concepts and allegorical pictures.

The theological structure of the Old Testament is largely an Hebraic mythology, influenced by the mythologies of preceding and contemporary peoples. Its ethical code is strikingly primordial, swift vengeance transcending the element of compassion or human sympathy. The spirit of reprisal is paramount, both in dealing with individuals and nations, and this same hectic passion for inflicting punishment was projected upon its deity—Jehovah. An ardor for direct and summary vengeance is the attribute of all mythological gods.

While the New Testament, through the benign influence of Jesus, sounds a more gentle note in man's relation with man, the entire theme represents a many-sided picture of rich symbolism in a dim, faraway background. This dream-like property is a powerful attraction to the primitive nature of modern man.

So it is that institutional religion still retains a potent influence by symbolically *taking man back into the past,* and offering him a paradise in the future. The first satisfies the primitive tendency toward regression, and the second the primitive desire of the ego for immortality. Those religions which are the richest in symbolism have attained the greatest measure of power and have been most successful in holding their following.

Oral demonstration in religion is another phase of emotionalism that vouchsafes an outlet for psychic pressure. Song, confession and public declaration of faith are the principal media of expression. Music is the most effective of all stimuli for readily awakening strong emotional response, either with respect to religious worship, martial combat or sensuality. Again, it will be noted that all of these are elemental expressions of the primitive personality.

That confession affords a means of relief of psychic or emotional tension is undeniable. The murderer experiences a profound relief when he has divulged his secret guilt, even though he is tormented by the knowledge of the law's retribution. Even the latter is less unbearable than the festering consciousness of unacknowledged guilt. The Catholic secures peace of mind through confession to his priest; the Protestant by unburdening his conscience in prayer.

In many sects, emotional outbursts are a regular part of the services. There are some important and well-known "shouting" sects, not to mention a host of smaller ones. No one would contend that there is any intellectual benefit derived from these demonstrations. The appeal is purely primi-

tive, and the response purely emotional. Nevertheless, to people whose lives are otherwise emotionally starved, the relief of psychic tension afforded by voluble religious expression fulfils a
fundamental need. The primitive personality receives at least a partial outlet for its constantly
accumulating energy.

Sometimes an example of effusive religious
ecstasy will be found that may be considered either
saintly and sublime, or dementia, depending upon
the historical period in which it is manifested.

Southey, in his *Life of Wesley,* instances one of
the most rapturous cases of conversion on record
—that of a young woman in her twentieth year,
a disciple of Wesley's, whom she called her "dear
and most honoured father in Christ." The change
in her condition began with a *"violent agony* of
about four hours' duration." "Then," said the
patient, "I began to feel the Spirit of God bearing witness with my spirit that I was born of God.
Oh, mighty, powerful, happy change! The love
of God was shed abroad in my heart, and a flame
kindled there with *pains so violent, yet so very
ravishing,* that my body was almost torn asunder.
I sweated; I trembled; I fainted; I sang. Oh, I
thought my head was a fountain of water. I was
dissolved in love. *My beloved is mine and I am
his.* He has all charms; he has ravished my heart;
he is my comforter, my friend, my all. He is now
in his garden feeding among the lilies. Oh, I am
sick of love. He is altogether lovely, the chiefest

among ten thousand. Oh, how Jesus fills, Jesus extends, Jesus overwhelms the soul in which He dwells.''

This declaration of faith is remarkable for more than the display of obviously sincere enthusiasm. It is a perfect example of symbolic picturization, with a pronounced erotic coloring, as must be plain to anyone who has made even the most superficial study of symbolism.

BIBLIOGRAPHY

SWISHER, W. S., *Religion and the New Psychology*, Boston, 1920.

JAMES, WILLIAM, *Varieties of Religious Experience*, New York.

CARPENTER, EDWARD, *Pagan and Christian Creeds*, New York, 1920.

FREUD, SIGMUND, *Totem and Taboo*, New York, 1918.

LAY, WILFRID, *Man's Unconscious Spirit*, New York, 1921.

FORLONG, J. G. R., *Rivers of Life or Faiths of Men*.

JENNINGS, HARGRAVE, *Phallicism*.

KNIGHT, PAYNE, *The Worship of Priapus*.

WESTROPP, HODDER M., *Primitive Symbolism*.

STONE, LEE A., *Phallic Symbolism*, ''The Urologic and Cutaneous Review,'' St. Louis, December, 1920.

JUNG, C. G., *Psychology of the Unconscious*, New York, 1917.

## CHAPTER XI

## THE CAVEMAN REBELS

It is proof of great thought to separate thought from habit.—CICERO.

THERE is a fundamental, restless, irrepressible urge that pervades the human organism, that characterizes the human being. It has been called the energetic constitution of man, the prime mover of human action. Freud has termed it the *libido;* Bergson, the *élan vital;* Jung the *horme.* It is essentially a *craving.* It is the craving for Life, for Love, for Action. Basically it is primitive, and it retains its elemental features at all times, although it is capable of great social adaptation, which has been called, for the want of a better term, *sublimation.* It is the spirit of the Caveman.

It expresses itself in every human being, normal and abnormal, but in widely diverging channels and in very uneven degrees of effectiveness. I have said that it is irrepressible, to which objection may be taken because of the conformity of the multitudes. As a matter of fact, it cannot be repressed. If the attempt is made at one point, it will break out in another. The spirit of conformity that is fostered is compensated for in the irrational attitudes and actions, and the pathology of everyday life.

Nietzsche, with his vision of the Superman, and his struggle—almost successful—to be one, called this human dynamic the "will-to-power." Alfred Adler refers to it as the "wish-to-be-above." It is both; it is the Ego.

## The Ego Urge

In order to understand the working of such an intangible, mysterious force as the ego, it is necessary to study its action under certain specific conditions. We cannot see electricity, but we can observe the operation of motors and machinery, we can visualize the arc and incandescent lights, and watch a great many other manifestations of the elusive electric current. So it is with the vital, invisible current—Life itself.

Adler's theory of organ inferiority and its physical compensation opens up vast possibilities for research in this domain. In considering Adler's hypothesis, it is well to bear in mind the functions of the autonomic nervous system and of the endocrine (ductless) glands, referred to in Chapter II.

Few people are born with or, if so, long retain, a perfectly adjusted organism. For example, we know that poor eyesight and defective hearing are commonplace. Countless numbers of people have weak hearts or bad digestions, and the number of other organic disturbances (trivial or serious) is limited only by the number of organs in the body.

What are the results of these defects or maladjustments? Nature is as resourceful as she is prolific. She is ever seeking to adapt, not to social conditions or ethical concepts, but to biological requirements. When some particular organ is defective, there is always a tendency—nature's effort to strike a new adjustment—for some other organ to develop a greater functional capacity to overcome the handicap to the body as a whole. Subnormal organs show more plasticity and adaptability than do normal organs.

This deviation from a normal physiological balance must of necessity affect the psyche, sometimes stimulating it to compensate in an intellectual or emotional way for the physical handicap; or, on the other hand, often adversely influencing the mental processes through fear or worry over the defect.

Janet and other distinguished neurologists of the old school have mentioned that the neurotic's sense of inferiority, which has been called a "sense of incompleteness," sought compensation in neurotic imaginings.

A study of the mechanistic factors of behavior shows that one of the prime effects of organ inferiority of any kind is to promote nervous activity. This increased nervous activity, if it is not vouchsafed an outlet for constructive, creative work, will turn within and work havoc in the form of a neurosis. It is this combination of circumstances, a defective organ and a highly charged nervous system, with great energetic capacity, that has been so conspicuous in the pathological history of genius. Subnormal organs, under the stimulation of the autonomic nervous system, and when augmented by compensatory activity of other organs or functions with which they are correlated, develop supernormal properties in the body as a whole.

In Chapter XV, it will be noted that the most representative geniuses in all fields of endeavor had suffered from pronounced physical defects of one sort or another, which reacted in the form of increased nervous energy. At least there were physical and psychic disabilities which were accompanied by great nervous energy. This excess of nerve force often found an outlet in eccentric or irrational actions—indeed, not infrequently in the form of insanity.

History records numerous cases of those who, steeled apparently by the struggle against physical handicap, have risen to heights of creative achievement. The irrepressible Caveman within will not tolerate a feeling of inferiority. There is always the tendency to compensate for any sort of weakness.

Some of the more commonplace forms of compensation are readily recognized. Little men walk erect; tall men stoop. There is the bravery of the physically small; the bragging of the timid; the washing mania of the immoral; the cheerfulness of the dying (tuberculosis psychosis) ; the patriotism of the unheroic. People with a weak stomach become interested in the nutritive values and digestive properties of foods, and frequently become expert on these subjects. Subnormal eyesight intensifies the visual psyche. An art school investigated by Adler showed a larger percentage of defective eyesight than any other gathering of young people.

Mozart had an imperfectly developed ear; Beethoven had otosclerosis, and finally became totally deaf. Demosthenes, Aristotle, Virgil and Lamb were among the stammerers. Homer, Timoleon and Milton were blind. Æsop was crippled in body. Alexander the Great, Caesar, St. Paul, Petrarch, Mohammed, Charles V, Napoleon, Dostoevsky, were a few of the great epileptics. Socrates, ungainly of limb and ugly of body, developed a wonderful mind. Byron was clubfooted. Epictetus, once a slave, was maimed in body but indomitable in spirit. De Quincey was large-headed and wizened-bodied. Charles Darwin did not know what it was to enjoy a day of good health for forty years. Laura Bridgman and Helen Keller, deaf, dumb and blind, achieved fame in spite of these formidable obstacles. The extraordinary imagination of Robert Louis Stevenson was developed at the expense of an ailing, tubercular body. Roosevelt transformed a frail physique into a human dynamo. Edison, defective in hearing, utilized his excessive energy in the domain of scientific achievement.

The ancients must have noted this tendency, as they attributed defects to some of their important mythological gods. Odin, chief of the Norse Gods, had one eye; Tyr, God of War, one hand; Vidar, slayer of the Wolf of Fenrer, was dumb. Vulcan, the Roman's God of Fire, was lame.

The reports of the Massachusetts Asylum for the Blind make mention of a female deaf and blind mute, Julia Brace, who had developed an extraordinary compensatory faculty in the sense of smell. Anyone whom she had met before she recognized by smell. She knew all of her acquaintances by the smell of their hands, and was able to perceive and distinguish odors that other persons could not detect. In sorting clothes that had come for the wash, she could distinguish those of each friend. If half a dozen strangers were present and each threw his glove into a hat, and the gloves were mixed, Julia would take them up and by means of smell alone, return them to their owners. She could also tell brothers and sisters by smell.

### Authority Complex

Just as every individual struggles against physical handicap, he likewise struggles against repressive factors in his environment. The reactions to the inhibitory forces of our environment are manifold in their scope, and produce paradoxical results.

Undue parental repression may result in stifling the initiative of a child, in which case the energetic force turns within and through introversion creates a neurosis; or, the exercise of unwise parental restrictions may turn the child into a confirmed, unreasonable rebel against any kind of authority.

In the first situation, the ego seeks an abnormal form of compensation through neurotic substitute gratification. In the second, there is an abnormal compensation because, although going in the right direction, the ego-urge has gone beyond all rational bounds. The original trend to rebelliousness was justified because it represents an attempt to resist an authority that threatens the development of the individual's personality. As a matter of fact, every living organism struggles to express itself, and resents suppression or repression.

The confirmed rebelliousness that degenerates into *negativism* is a chronic resistance due to an authority complex. It is useless, however, to condemn it without an insight into its genesis. And an understanding of it brings to us a realization that, after all, it is the ego-urge striving to be felt. As this striving is essential to the development of personality and character, the tendency is sound at bottom, but it has simply got out of all control of the individual, whom it dominates.

Examples may be noted of persons of creative

genius who have been profoundly influenced by an authority complex. The positive trend in these cases is exceptional. Instead of nursing their complexes on the sour milk of futility and disruption, they have gained a certain amount of ego-satisfaction by turning them into constructive revolutionary channels.

Wagner is a distinguished example of the artist who turns his rebellous fervour into imperishable music. Voltaire, Schopenhauer, Nietzsche, Carlyle, Ibsen, were incurable iconoclasts who have enriched the world of philosophy and letters. A whole school of Russian writers, embittered by the blanket oppression of the Czars, which had permeated the whole social atmosphere of their country, has given us a remarkable literature that cannot be duplicated in any other nation.

Perhaps no creative neurotic offers a better illustration of the authority complex and the resultant struggle against an over-powering feeling of inferiority than Strindberg. From childhood, Strindberg was obsessed by the idea of his fancied inferiority, and his life represented a series of desperate efforts to climb out of this estate. So confirmed was he in his obsession, because of the powerful influence the complex exerted upon him, that all his marvelous creative power was futile to lift him above his fears. He succumbed finally to the Nemesis of inferiority that had haunted him from the beginning; dying with "the cross before his eyes and hate in his heart,"—the cross, the everlasting symbol of inability to master an earthly life, and hate, the negation of all emotional value.

The tragedy of the typical neurotic's attempt to realize his goal of superiority is that the goal is a fictitious or unreal one. He squanders incalculable energy in attempting to attain it. He is driven toward it by the impetus of his unfulfilled (i.e., unfulfillable) desires. His goal is as useless as it is vague and impossible. If attained, it would benefit neither himself nor anyone else. True to neurotic form, he is on the wrong track. The only relief possible is through insight into, and reintegration of, his unconscious mental processes, which will then enable him to direct his ideas and attitudes toward reality.

### Radicalism

The radical is a person whose ego rebels against one or several socially organized repressions. The term radicalism, however, is popularly associated with any movement that runs counter to the dominant factor in the social organization. In the days when the Church held temporal supremacy, radicalism was directed principally against the abuses and restrictions of ecclesiasticism. The radicals of the Middle Ages were those who ached under the ecclesiastical ban on unauthorized teachings and ideas. Today the most thoroughgoing free thinker is not considered radical if his political and economic opinions are orthodox.

Immediately after the church's decline in temporal power, the true radicals were political dissenters who protested against the absolutism of kings and other hereditary monarchs. They advocated the cause of the growing commercial class, the bourgeoisie, who were finally triumphant, barring some remnants of feudalism that remained in Europe up to the time of the World War. Today one may be the staunchest kind of bourgeois democrat and still escape the stigma of radicalism if he is a conformist in his economic ideas.

At the present time, the radical is the advocate of industrial democracy. The dominant power of contemporary society lies with the industrial-economic régime, so support of this institution becomes the criterion of orthodoxy.

The principal point in this discussion is that the same psychological factor that made the ecclesiastic radical later made the political radical, and finally the typical economic radical. They all rebelled against the dominant system of their time, because they associated it (unconsciously for the most part) with an unbearable authority.

It may be that there has been a rare rebel in every epoch who reasoned his course out by the cold, dispassionate method of absolute logic. Even the rarest of these, I believe, has drawn in part upon his unconscious memories of a soul-revolting authority in childhood.

Undoubtedly, the most logical, dispassionate, coldly calculating rebel of the present epoch is Lenin. Both his friends and his enemies, by direct statement or implication, admit this. Whether acclaimed a devil or a saint, there is a general agreement on this point. But to understand the psychology of Lenin, we must consider that, although coming from a family of the Russian nobility, he has been a rebel from his early youth. I have never come across any description of his father, but can readily imagine him to have been an iron-willed despot of the characteristic Russian nobleman type. Perhaps even Lenin inherited the qualities which he grew to hate in the personality of his father. And then, while still in his teens, he saw his older brother, also a confirmed rebel, fall a gallows victim of the Czar's hangmen. Is it not probable that the emotional reaction of this shock has left its indelible imprint on the mentality of Lenin, and that it has contributed to his determination to smash all that he associated with the old order?

The development of modern industry, with its constant trend toward specialization, is directly responsible, from a psychological viewpoint, for acute outbreaks of the ego-urge in the way of radical agitation. Wholesale production does not satisfy the instinct for workmanship, contrivance or constructiveness. The desire for individual

achievement is seldom fulfilled, in modern industry, so that by the denial of one of the fundamental
cravings of the ego, there is prepared a fertile
background for discontent. This is true irrespec-
tive of the question of wages and other working
conditions, although these of course are vital
factors in the industrial relations. The point is,
even were all other working conditions ideal, there
would be radical discontent if the creative instinct
were denied an outlet.

In the old days of handicraft, when the work-
man made his product from start to finish, instead
of specializing on a single part or a single operation, he was able to express his originality and
personality. This opportunity for creative effort
fulfilled a psychological need which is lost to
modern industry. It is the problem of any society
that can claim to be fundamentally sound to overcome this defect by substituting some constructive outlet for the creative instinct.

In this country extreme economic radicalism is
epitomized in the Industrial Workers of the
World. This opens up a vast subject that cannot
even be outlined here. It may be suggested, however, that I. W. W.'ism is a result of some sinister
cause. It is an effect that should be traced to its
roots, and not blindly suppressed, leaving the cor-
roding cause to remain. The late Professor Carleton H. Parker, who has made the most extensive
disinterested investigation into the I. W. W. problem, said that it can be profitably viewed only as

a psychological by-product of the neglected childhood of industrial America. He further stated,
"There will be neither permanent peace nor pros-
perity in our country till the revolt-bases of the
I. W. W. are removed, and till that is done the
I. W. W. remains an unfortunately valuable symptom of a diseased industrialism."

No less an authority than Dr. Jacques Loeb
(*Comparative Physiology of the Brain*) has
stressed the importance of the instinct of workmanship, and the evil results of denying it an
adequate outlet. He summed it up in these words:
". . . Lawyers, criminologists and philosophers
frequently imagine that only want makes man
work. This is an erroneous view. We are instinctively forced to be active in the same way as ants
and bees. The instinct of workmanship would be
the greatest source of happiness if it were not
for the fact that our present social and economic
organization allows only a few to satisfy this instinct. . . . *The greatest happiness in life* can be
obtained only if *all instincts,* that of workmanship
included, can be maintained at a certain *optimal
intensity.* But while it is certain that the individual can ruin or diminish the value of its life by
a one-sided development of its instincts, e.g. dis-
sipation, it is at the same time true that the
*economic and social conditions can ruin or di-
minish the value of life for a great number of
individuals.* It is no doubt true that in our own
present social and economic conditions more than

ninety per cent. of human beings lead an existence whose value is far below what it should be."

## *Conservatism*

The authority complex is also the psychological foundation of conservatism. Unlike the instance of radicalism, there is lacking the resistance to the basic motive. Instead of generating an intense conflict, with its consequent rebelliousness, it promotes a feeling of dependence on someone or thing whom it associates with parental authority. This form of reaction is particularly deplorable when it robs the subject of all reasonable confidence in himself. He (or she) must have someone to lean upon. He depends upon others for his opinions. He lacks initiative, although he talks much about his plans, which never materialize. He tends to follow the crowd, instead of acting as a thinking individual. He becomes essentially a unit of the crowd instead of a real personality. The significance of this is demonstrated in Chapter XIII.

It is a fact of mass psychology that the inhibitions of childhood, as personified in parental authority, should be continued in the authority of organized society. Everywhere, we are fenced in by "Don'ts." As a matter of fact, the great majority of people expect them, and would be quite at sea without this constant expression of authority to look up to.

Those who most sincerely respect and uphold this situation are grown-up children, called adults, who carry about in the Unconscious a dominating parent-image, or authority complex. Unable to come to any rational decision by way of independent thinking on their own account, they always look to some superior authority when in doubt, as the child does to its father.

To the child, the father, whether wise or ignorant, is the personification of wisdom and strength. Indeed, the ignorant parent is apt to use his physical strength in lieu of wisdom.

The adult child finds his fancied protection, not in attempting to reason out the *why,* and *wherefore,* and *whence* of problems that confront him, but in leaning on the strength of superior authority. This he recognizes in established institutions —the state and all its subdivisions, the church, and, to a degree that he does not consciously realize, the newspaper he reads and frequently ridicules.

In the hysteria of war-times, the reaction of the authority complex is particularly notable. It was a former Attorney General of the United States, I believe, who issued the edict early in the Great War which was placarded in public places all over the country: *"Obey the law and keep your mouth shut!"* The elegance of this phraseology is exceeded only by its edifying purport. It would be difficult to imagine popularizing anything so crude except under the influence of the war spirit—and among grown-up children.

These soul-stirring words, to many an adult-child, carried the connotation of parental authority. The brusque warning might be laughed at as a joke, or slightly resented as an infringement on a citizen's right to express himself, but nevertheless, to the great majority, it symbolized the voice of the Great Father—the State.

The conservatism that intelligently selects and retains that which has proven its worth in human experience is a truly conserving force. A different kind of "conservatism" is the indiscriminate stand-pat-ism of the individual dominated by an authority complex. To this ·universal type, authority is summed up in precedent. What *is,* must be right. All the approved institutions, with their long line of precedent, speak with authority which must not be questioned. This kind of conservative is "a man who believes that nothing should ever be done for the first time."

An intimate knowledge of our psychic operations is bound to diminish the primitive strength of the herd-instinct, and to develop individuality and self-reliance. By dissipating the parent complex, we loosen the strangle hold of authority, and pave the way for a fuller expression of the creative will. This irradiation will do much to relieve us of our repressions, taboos and shackling fears. It will be a powerful influence in converting destructive impulses, and in freeing the dynamic faculties of both the unconscious and conscious mind.

## BIBLIOGRAPHY

ADLER, ALFRED, *Organ Inferiority and Its Psychic Compensation,* Nervous and Mental Disease Monograph Series No. 24.

ADLER, ALFRED, *The Neurotic Constitution,* New York, 1917.

BJERRE, POUL, *The History and Practice of Psychoanalysis,* Boston, 1916.

PARKER, CARLETON H., *The Casual Laborer and other Essays,* New York, 1920.

VEBLEN, THORSTEIN, *The Instinct of Workmanship,* New York, 1918.

TEAD, ORDWAY, *Instincts in Industry,* Boston, 1919.

TROTTER, W., *Instincts of the Herd in Peace and War,* New York, 1919.

SANGER, MARGARET, *Woman and the New Race,* New York, 1920.

SANGER. MARGARET, *The Pivot of Civilization,* New York, 1922.

# CHAPTER XII

# THE CAVEMAN'S HALTED DEVELOPMENT

Conscious professed ideals are as straws in the wind;
the unconscious or concealed ideals are the real forces
that govern mankind.—GILBERT MURRAY.

IN recognition of the extent, and apparent
increase, of mental subnormality, Professor
William McDougall begins his recent, much-dis-
cussed work, *Is America Safe for Democracy?*
with this startling observation: "As I watch the
American nation speeding gaily, with invincible
optimism, down the road to destruction, I seem
to be contemplating the greatest tragedy in the
history of mankind."

A number of volumes, and many contributions
to periodicals, have appeared within the past few
years, dealing with the problems of low mental
age among adults, as disclosed by army statistics
during the war. Most of these works are of value
chiefly in bringing to public attention a very deplorable condition, and the wide discussion which
has followed may help to a great extent in finding
and applying a remedy. It seems to me that the
general tendency has been to over-emphasize the
genetic side of the question and to minimize the

environmental factors.  In making this statement,
I do not wish it presumed that I am under-rating
the importance of hereditary qualities.  I merely
wish to have it brought home that there are *two*
sides to the question, and *both* must have adequate consideration.


### Army Mental Tests

In order to appreciate the extent of mental
deficiency and illiteracy among the adult population of the country, we can do no better than
review some of the data collected by the Army
authorities during the war.  That there is a distinction between illiteracy and mental deficiency
is, of course, obvious, although both are in the
nature of social liabilities, as well as personal
handicaps.

It was the intention that the tests should be not
at all a barometer of knowledge, and not of a
kind to give much scope to such mental training
as is developed at school.  The results were calculated to represent innate mental ability—*intelligence.*

The army intelligence examination was given
to 1,726,966 men, of whom 41,000 were officers.
Nearly thirty per cent. of the 1,556,011 men for
whom statistics were available when Messrs.
Yoakum and Yerkes published their report, were
found to be unable to ''read and understand news-

papers and write letters home,"[1] and were given a special examination prepared for illiterates.

An explanation of the mental ratings for the various classifications, and the respective percentages of those who took the tests, follows:

A. *Very superior intelligence.* This grade was ordinarily reached by only four and one-half per cent. of a draft quota. It was composed of men of marked intellectuality, with the ability to make a superior record in college or university.

B. *Superior intelligence.* Less exceptional than that represented by "A," and was obtained by nine per cent. of the draft. Men of this group are capable of making an average record in college.

C+. *High average intelligence.* This group included about sixteen and one-half per cent. of the draft. Cannot do so well as "B," but contained some men with capacity for leadership and power to command.

C. *Average intelligence.* Included about twenty-five per cent. of drafted men. These men are rarely capable of graduating from a high school. They are of a grade that is said to make "excellent privates" in the army. Their mental age may be put at about fourteen.

C—. *Low average intelligence.* These men made up about twenty per cent. of the draft. Although below average intelligence, they are "usually good privates and satisfactory in work of a

[1] *Army Mental Tests,* page 12.

routine nature.'' Mental age probably not below twelve.

D. *Inferior intelligence.* Included about fifteen per cent. of the draft. Are usually slow in learning, but likely to make fair soldiers. It is unsafe to expect these, or those of grades "D—" and "E" to read intelligently or to understand·written directions.

D— and E. *Very inferior intelligence.* Comprised about ten per cent. of the soldiers. The majority of these men were below the mental age of ten—some were discovered with a mental age as low as two or three, and were being passed upon for sending to France in 1918.

Between April 27th and November 30, 1918, 7749 men (0.5 per cent.) were reported for discharge by psychological examiners because of mental inferiority. The recommendations for assignment to labor battalions because of low-grade intelligence, numbered 9871 (0.6 + per cent.). 9432 (0.6 + per cent.) were recommended for assignment to development battalions for further observation to determine if there might be ways of using them in the Army.

During this same seven-months' interval, there were reported 4700 men with a mental age below seven years; 7762 between seven and eight years; 14,566 between eight and nine years; 18,581 between nine and ten years. This gives a total of 45,653 men under ten years of age mentally. The authors of *Army Mental Tests* consider it extremely improbable that many of these individuals were worth what it cost the government to maintain, equip and train them for military service.

Assuming that the drafted men were a fair sample of the mental development of our 100,-000,000 population, it means that forty-five millions, nearly one-half of the whole population, have the mental capacity of a normal twelve-year-old child, and that only thirteen and one-half per cent. possess superior intelligence.

Turning for the moment from mental inferiority to illiteracy, as late as June 17, 1921, in an address at Sea Girt, N. J., under the auspices of the Military Order of the World War, General Pershing was reported in the press to have stated: "The illiteracy of a high percentage of the young manhood of America is a disgrace to any nation . . . "

### Emotional Immaturity

Aside from mental age, which is subject to arrestment at various levels, there is also an emotional progression that may be halted at almost any stage¡ instead of arriving at a well-rounded maturity. There is often a discrepancy between the intellectual and the emotional levels in the same individual. In too many cases, they are both below normal, but it can readily be understood that one reacts upon the other and influences it accordingly.

From the emotional side, which indicates the domination of unconscious ideas and urges, it has been proposed that there are five ages of man. These are not hard and fast classifications, but are arranged as a tentative working basis for study and discussion. As a matter of fact, there may be any number of graduations between the lowest and the highest.

In infancy, the emotional age is characterized by absolute dependence upon the mother or her substitute. Ferenczi, the Hungarian psychologist, who has thrown much light upon this subject, has divided infancy into the following periods: (1) unconditional omnipotence; (2) magical-hallucinatory omnipotence; (3) omnipotence by the help of magic gestures; (4) omnipotence by magic thoughts and magic words.

After infancy there follows the first emotional age of childhood, ranging from about four to seven years, during which the repressive influences of the social environment make a very deep and permanent impression on the child.

The second childhood age, covering the period from seven to the beginning of puberty, is characterized by physical growth and muscular development. It is also in this stage that the child begins to detach itself from its parents by forming attachments outside the family circle.

The pubescent age runs along from twelve to

seventeen. The first figure is the average earliest age for girls, and the second the average latest age for boys. It is at this age that the sexual side of the adolescent rapidly completes its development, and the reactions of this climacteric situation on the whole organism, physically, mentally and spiritually, are very pronounced.

The fifth and final emotional age, which is reached, without any question of doubt, by a minority of people only, is that of well-rounded adulthood. Normally, it signifies the completion of the evolution of the emotions. In all other cases, the maladjustments of the emotional mechanism, which had their origin in the preceding ages, may express themselves in the most aggravating forms.

Very often a high order of mental capacity will be accompanied by emotional under-development. A man may be a success in his business, having overcome many formidable obstacles, and still, because of some unfavorable situation in his early life, suffer from a stoppage in the unfolding of his emotional nature. This condition is invariably represented by a desire of the victim to return, symbolically, to the stage at which his emotions became fixed. His ideals become more and more centered on emotional stimuli that he should normally have lived through and outgrown.

Many petty sadists, not to speak of the more extreme types, who inflict their cruelties on those over whom they have authority, are examples of persons suffering from arrested emotional development. They may be keen of mind, and apparently mature, but they are emotionally chained to a primitive, preadolescent level that would be normal for childhood. They are characterized by a feverish spirit of restlessness and dissatisfaction. With their adult physique and relatively mature mental development, they are living paradoxes. One side of the Caveman in particular is constantly cropping out. People of this type need psychic re-education. An insight into their psychical processes is invariably helpful. These cases are among the most hopeful because they have the intelligence required to grasp the situation when it is disclosed to them.

The "hoodlum," on the other hand, is an individual who has grown to physical maturity and remains at a low *mental* and *emotional* level. He is a man in body, but a child, that is, a *savage*, in mind and character.

Children who pass through the evolving stages of youth without the love, attention and care that should be the birthright of every child, invariably suffer from emotional starvation. And there are literally millions of children who, because of the family's extreme poverty, or sickness or other misfortune befalling one or both of the parents, reach physical and sometimes mental adulthood with the invisible chains of an emotionally unfulfilled childhood drawing them back to a chapter of life they have been denied, and which they cannot now obtain.

Many of these people may meet with material success, some in a very substantial way, but they are spiritual failures in the adult world. While society, seeing only the material aspects, may not realize the drawback, their families and the wives, in particular, are the ones who face the consequences and suffer the penalties of a fate, of which all concerned are the unknowing victims.

While a comparatively few of those so handicapped have surmounted the obstacles of an emotionally starved childhood and risen to distinguished adulthood notwithstanding, who will say that there are not vast numbers that have found the terrific handicap of the past too great to overcome. Careful observation will disclose, too, that it is not always the intellectually favored who succeed in a material way, but rather those who have a fair mind and the stronger physical constitution. Surrounded by a barrier of crushing physical odds, the superior intellect, so frequently associated with a more sensitive and delicately balanced nervous system, is all too often vanquished by the competitor of coarser texture.

The history of the greatest material successes of this age is not a record of the triumph of the finest minds, signifying nobility of character, conscientiousness, social and personal honesty; instead, especially in laying their foundations, it has been for the most part a sordid chronicle of chicanery, craft, cunning, trickery in competition, political debauchery and ruthless exploitation.

### Heredity versus Environment

There seems to be a tendency on the part of academic psychologists, theoretical eugenists and anthropologists, in their concentration on some specialized study, usually the absorbing subject of heredity, to minimize, and often to overlook entirely, the question of environment. It may be that controversies over the relative importance of heredity and environment are futile because the two factors are so essentially unlike that comparison is impossible. Well then, we shall not discuss their *relative* importance. But there still remains the fact that there are two factors to be *considered*, each on its own account and in its relation to the other.

A writer on eugenics has disposed of the tremendously important social problems (which constitute environment) in the most off-hand way by this naïve declaration: "A mentally strong man in an unfortunate environment is self-impelled to get out of it and into one which matches his powers."

If a "strong mind" were a disincarnated mechanism, there might be some merit to this contention. But we must remember that a strong and even brilliant mind makes its advent into this world in a mortal body that is subject to all the warping, twisting and degrading influences of a pernicious environment. And as the "mind" is no less a part of the human organism than the "body," they are equally influenced, for good or ill, by environmental factors.

. In contrast to the fallacious extreme of virtually ignoring environmental influences, let us consider the statement of Dr. Morton Prince, the eminent psychiatrist: "That our points of view, attitudes of mind, sentiments, and the meaning which ideas have for us are determined by the experiences of life and are, therefore, *acquired,* can scarcely be traversed." [2]

Now, as man, intellectually and emotionally, is simply a bundle of opinions, attitudes and sentiments, which may direct his whole life along positive and constructive, or negative and destructive, lines, it can readily be seen that environment is of very fundamental importance.

The mind that is most responsive to sensory stimuli and is capable of higher development is a plastic material that may also be worked upon by the blighting agencies of a soul-crucifying environment. Thus the slums always have produced, and will continue to produce, social misfits, incompetents and criminals with fatalistic certainty.

Society's responsibility for criminality has been summarized by Professor Calkins in these words: "The criminal is not merely an individual delin-

[2] *The Journal of Abnormal Psychology*, Vol. XI, April, 1916.

quent; he is a social product. And society is chargeable with some portion of his guilt. If he is sent to prison, then we should all be sent to prison with him, but since this is impracticable the least we can do is to try to restore him. He is properly the object not of retribution, but of redemption.''

From certain highly esteemed sources, fearful for the future, there issues a feverish clamour for a revival of racial strength by the dual method of stimulating the birth-rate of the "fit" and ending the propagation of the "unfit." It would seem logical, before agitating an increase in human numbers from any social group, first to assure every child that is born into the world "fit" a chance to develop into a racial asset. Only too often the rough edges of society crush indiscriminately the fit and unfit, unless a kindly disposed fate drops them into a favourable environment.

And it should be equally self-evident that accessibility of contraceptive information to married people of the less effective social groups would contribute materially to the racial welfare. There appears to be a feeling among the theoretical eugenists that the excessive birth-rate among the less fortunately situated is due to carelessness, or is even deliberate. As a matter of fact, everyone who has had the least contact with this situation knows that in the overwhelming majority of cases, it is *helplessness,* which may eventually sink into the inertia of hopelesness.

The burden of excessive progeny among those economically handicapped is in itself conducive to "unfitness." It results in a disintegration of the family morale, to the moral, intellectual and physical detriment of its individual units. So it will be seen that the evils of racial degeneration, which are reflected in a low mental and emotional age, are bound up with prolificacy in any socially unfavorable environment.

It is true, as the heredity specialists declare, that oak trees will come only from an oak stock. But we know that a certain environment will warp an oak, making it comparatively valueless; and that a continuation of unfavorable environmental factors will dwarf its line so that we have a literal scrub oak. And the best of human material, subjected to the deteriorating forces of an unpropitious environment, will degenerate into a scrub stock.

In stressing the influences of environment, I do not wish to imply that I am out of sympathy with the fundamental principles of eugenics, or that I underrate the magnificent work of Galton and his followers. Their contribution to human progress is an invaluable one. Nevertheless, there is a tendency on the part of certain influential writers in the eugenics movement to present a thoroughly one-sided picture of the racial problem.

Mr. Edward Thomas in his book, *Industry, Emotions and Unrest,* refers to tests made at the University of Pennsylvania's Psychological Clinic for children suspected of being mentally defective, which indicated that more than ninety per cent. of the children brought to it regained a normal development when placed in proper care.

Commenting on the observation that among children of orphan institutions generally, nearly half of the children in large orphanages are seriously defective in brain power and that the older ones are more affected than the others, Mr. Thomas was informed by a psychologist that probably few of these children are really defective. He believed that they had not been co-ordinated with the conventions of everyday life.

These children, deprived of the therapeutic balm of love and denied the opportunities for mental unfoldment that would be present in some degree in a normal family life, are subnormal from environmental pressure. And as they grow up into physical adulthood, the mentality becomes crystallized and remains static at some age-level of childhood.

Even in great numbers of homes, because of the neurotic tendencies and lack of insight on the part of the parents, children are subjected to conditions that tend to prevent the full development of their mental possibilities and emotional nature.

The genetic authorities are doubtless quite correct in reminding us that education cannot in-

crease the intellectual potentialities or capacities.
But that is only half the story. A fact equally
important is that the opportunities must be *available* in order to assure the development of the
existent potentialities and capacities. Furthermore, the possibilities of education are not realized in the "cram and emetic" process (to quote
Saleeby) of prevailing pedagogic methods.

Education, in reality, is the development of
the faculties through *expression* of the personality and is bound up with every phase of life.
It is the *art of living*. It begins at birth and ends
either at death or with the fossilization of the
intellect—and only too often it is the latter.

As schools, with few exceptions, work on children in the mass (grades) and prescribe a uniform curriculum for all pupils within any given
class or grade, little or no allowance is made for
personal idiosyncrasies or expressions of individuality. Now and then an exceptionally enlightened teacher is found who, on his or her own
initiative, makes the fullest allowances possible,
under the restrictions of the pedagogic system,
for the expression and development of the individual qualities of the pupil.

But as education does not begin or end in
school, and is not confined to the class room during the school-attending period, the home life and
all the influences of the community play their part
in developing or warping the mind of the child.
In a sense, however, the school is typical of all

these various influencing factors, inasmuch as it represents the dominant spirit of *conformity*.

Children who do not conform are locally and institutionally damned. They are considered failures in school and misfits in the community. More often than not, they will be found among the intellectual pioneers of the morrow.[3] He was a profound student of human nature who observed: "Whoso would be a *man*, must be a non-conformist."

Dr. Saleeby has epitomized the failure of the prevailing educational institutions in the following comment: "A genius was educated at Eton, and we say that Eton produced him. The truth is, of course, that Eton failed to destroy him. (One says Eton for convenience, but the name of any accepted school will do.)"

And to avoid misunderstanding, I again repeat and emphasize that the schools are not singled

[3] "Many children who became great men had been regarded at school as bad, wild, or silly; but their intelligence appeared as soon as the occasion offered, or when they found the true path of their genius. It was thus with Thiers, Pestalozzi, Wellington, Du Guesclin, Goldsmith, Burns, Balzac, Fresnel, Dumas *père*, Humboldt, Sheridan, Boccaccio, Pierre Thomas, Linnæus, Volta, Alfieri. Thus Newton, meditating on the problems of Kepler, often forgot the orders and commissions given him by his mother; and while he was the last in his class, he was very clever in making mechanical playthings. Walter Scott, who also showed badly at school, was a wonderful story-teller. Gustave Flaubert was the very opposite of a phenomenal child. It was only with extreme difficulty that he succeeded in learning to read. His mind, however, was already working, for he composed little plays which he could not write, but which he represented alone, playing the different personages, and improvising long dialogues."— O. Lombroso.

out as lone offenders, but are used merely as an illustration that is typical of our approved social institutions.

## *Imitative Behavior*

Another factor that must be taken into consideration—a psychological one—is the universal proclivity of children, from the time of their earliest observation, consciously and unconsciously to imitate the actions, attitudes and expressions of their parents and others with whom they come in contact. A bright child reared in a home or community environment wherein there are mental defectives will imitate some of the peculiar idiosyncrasies of these people until they become ingrained into its personality.

The most promising children raised in an atmosphere of mental and emotional poverty must inevitably fail to achieve a high degree of mental development or maturity of emotional evolution, unless some happy, haphazard circumstance should intervene to offset the handicap.

The kinks of character that are produced in the formative period by an extremely faulty environment result in a lack of mental and moral stamina that the best of heredity cannot always overcome or outgrow.

Besides the more extreme cases of subnormal mentality that may be classified as, or border on, a pathological condition, regressions to childhood

mental levels are among the most common of all
psychological phenomena. As a matter of fact,
the psychic and emotional ties that connect us
with our childhood are so strong that they are
continually drawing us back. Only the vigilance
of the intellect and rational processes interferes
with these regressions.

Political convictions, religious beliefs and other
ideas that we absorb from our early environment
are notoriously impervious to reason or argument. We tend to adhere to the traditional faiths
of our childhood, and often do not care to discuss
them—only to *assert* them.

The man or woman who is forever judging
situations by the inflexible estimate of what "dear
mother" or "poor father" would do under the
circumstances, is demonstrating his or her childhood mental level. Things are appraised in the
light of childhood reminiscence instead of in their
relation to the present. Reality is disregarded in
favour of a childish, or even infantile, attitude.

As a result of these childhood barriers, and
their automatic influences over our judgments, we
have developed an intensive system of "rationalization." Logical reasoning on abstract subjects
is rare, and most rare of all is the inductive
method of analysis—i.e., classifying a series of
known facts and reasoning from them up to general principles; instead, preconceived notions and
ideas are supported by building up under them
an elaborate structure of justification, which may

be made to fit any conclusion. The average mind, fettered by certain childhood limitations, is satisfied with this inverted method—the antithesis of actual reasoning. One can justify any decision or opinion he may hold, because he has "reasoned" it out. This is a very convenient arrangement, because it enables one to retain the mental slothfulness of childhood, and still pose as a rational adult.

When Francis Bacon was grappling with medieval scholasticism three hundred years ago, he found this type of mind supreme, even dominating the so-called scientific and intellectual fields of that time. The two kinds of fallacies he had to combat were: "The proneness to support a preconceived opinion by affirmative instances, neglecting the opposing cases, and the tendency to generalize from an insufficient number of observations; the other type of errors being this—arising from the influence of mere words over the mind."

There have been great strides made since 1620 when Bacon gave to the world his *Novum Organum* — the thought-provoking instrument which proved to be the key that unlocked the door to the modern sciences. Under this impetus, the accurate sciences, physics, chemistry, technology, etc. developed into the industrial age. The so-called social sciences, however, have lagged behind. As it is these which constitute the educational, cultural, religious, political and ideological influences, much of the prevailing irrationality may be traced to anachronistic modes of thought emanating from this source.

Technological problems are studied and solved by the methods of positive science. Social problems are still left to speculative philosophies that are permeated with the decadent remnants of medievalism, but slightly disguised under a new terminology. Count Alfred Korzybski's valuable work, *The Manhood of Humanity*, already cited, throws a flood of light on this subject. Our whole social organization at present encourages, aids and abets mental subnormality.

## BIBLIOGRAPHY

McDougall, William, *Is America Safe for Democracy?* New York, 1921.

Yoakum, Clarence, and Robert M. Yerkes, *Army Mental Tests*, New York, 1920.

Terman, Lewis M., *The Measurement of Intelligence*, New York, 1916.

Terman, Lewis M., *Intelligence of School Children*, New York, 1919.

Goddard, H. H., *Human Efficiency and Levels of Intelligence*, Princeton, 1920.

Ballard, Philip Boswood, *Mental Tests*, London, 1920.

Evans, Elida, *The Problem of the Nervous Child*, New York, 1920.

Thomas, Edward, *Industry, Emotion and Unrest*, New York, 1920.

# CHAPTER XIII

## THE CAVEMAN BREAKS LOOSE

> Every human being has two personalities: an archaic,
> primitive, childlike, unadapted personality, and a modern,
> sophisticated, adult, and, to all appearances, adapted per-
> sonality.—ANDRÉ TRIDON.

THE intellectual and emotional immaturity of
a large section of the adult population is closely
allied to the tendency of the Caveman to break
loose—resulting in various manifestations of the
mob spirit. This lack of personal stability is
recognized in the etymology of the word "mob,"
which philologists tell us is the first syllable of
*mobile vulgus,* meaning vulgar or fickle people.

It might be assumed from this that all mobs are
up-wellings of the lower strata of society. There
is no doubt but what the term had its origin in
the contempt of the old aristocracy for the masses.
As a matter of fact, however, any group or class
of society as at present constituted is quite capable
of supplying effective mob material.[1]

The three requisites to convert any crowd into
a mob are emotionalism, lack of rational dis-

---

[1] "Any class may behave and think as a crowd—in fact it usually
does so in so far as its class interests are concerned."—Everett
Dean Martin, *The Behavior of Crowds.*

crimination (both of which are assured in practically every crowd) and some object of popular antipathy that is capable of turning the aroused feelings into mass action. In other words, every crowd is a potential mob.

The ethics of established social practices, under the influence of the mob spirit, fade away like so much vapor. Life may be taken, property destroyed—it is a gratification of the archaic desires within; a release of the psychic tension and suppressed emotions, a momentary return to the crude, primitive life of the Caveman.

The question of the specific motive in the analysis of mob psychology is of secondary importance; in fact, only a side issue. As the mob *feels* and *acts,* but does *not reason,* the feeling may be aroused either by some unbearable oppression, or by a lamentable prejudice. Spontaneous mob manifestations are invariably the result of the latter. Planned or organized mobs may be due to either prejudice or oppression. While mobs do not think, but turn blind emotionalism into precipitate action, their leaders in the case of an organized mob are apt to display much sagacity.

A mob may be animated by some age-old oppression, such as was the case with the mob which battered down the Bastille, or by a flagrant injustice, as was the case with the organized mob which had its celebrated Tea Party in Boston Harbor; or it may equally be motivated by an overbearing popular prejudice, as was the mob which destroyed

Lovejoy's printing press, and finally killed the determined Abolitionist; or the anti-Semitic fanatics of Georgia who murdered Leo Frank; the anti-I. W. W.ites who hung crippled Frank Little near Butte City; or the Colorado worthies who kidnapped Kate Richards O'Hare, the talented and eloquent speaker of a dissenting political party.

### Mass and Class Mobs

After our analysis of various anti-social manifestations of the Unconscious, as in dreams and other states in which our primitive nature asserts itself, it is interesting to note Mr. Everett Dean Martin's conclusion regarding the psychology of a crowd (potential mob) in his recent excellent work, *The Behavior of Crowds,* viz.: "My thesis is that *the crowd-mind is a phenomenon which should best be classed with dreams, delusions and various forms of automatic behavior.*"

Mr. Martin, too, maintains that the irresponsible behavior of the crowd is not limited to the masses, for he says that the cry of the Russian Revolution, " 'All power to the Soviets,' is peculiar neither to Russia nor to the working class. Such in spirit is the cry of every crowd, for every crowd is, psychologically considered, a soviet."

There are mass mobs, class mobs, college mobs, professional mobs, strike mobs, military mobs, national mobs, and others that could readily be classified. When a nation becomes hypnotized by an obsessive idea, as Germany was, it is a national mob. Regardless of the progress made in the technological sciences, there is the same psychological atmosphere nationally that animates the smaller crowd.

And considering the emotional nature and rational development of mankind generally, any nation might easily fall into the same delusion when the influence of all the mediums of popular propaganda, like the press, moving pictures, social organizations, political practices, economic pressure, etc., is employed to encourage people to behave and think as crowds. Even the schools and other educational, including religious, institutions contribute toward this end, by inculcating the idea of *uniformity of thought and action* (so typical of the crowd), instead of stimulating independent intellectual pursuit and critical self-analysis. The warnings of the greatest philosophers from Socrates ("look within thyself") to Emerson (urging *self*-reliance) have been ignored, and so everyone is required to jump into a strait-jacket of intellectual conformity.

When Liebknecht refused to conform to the intellectual goosestep of the German Junkers, and when Harden, in a lesser way, defied the national mob spirit of his country, we applauded their courageous actions. But when an individual in our own midst hesitated to follow the crowd, or suggested a little objective analysis of our methods and aims, we showed a vindictiveness which surpassed that faced by Liebknecht or Harden.

The frequency with which our state legislative bodies and the national congress pass hysterical legislation amply demonstrates the mob spirit at work in these august groups. The emotional outbursts that respond to a display of verbal pyrotechnics in almost any high-class gathering exposes the Caveman under a thin veneer of culture and broadcloth.

Le Bon, the French psychologist, avers that a crowd is not merely a gathering of people. It is primarily *a state of mind*. It represents a law of mental unity. And the quality of this state of mind, characteristically, seems to gravitate to the level of the lowest intelligence of the individual unit. This is because any higher rational expression or intellectual protest is lost in the current of primitive feeling. The obsessive idea of the crowd mind· is *compliance*. It follows with mechanical unanimity its single-tracked course of action, and will throttle without compunction any digression from the set course of the crowd spirit.

It is significant that the humanists, realists, pragmatists, throughout history have received scant consideration. Thinkers like Socrates, Protagoras, Epictetus, Bacon, Swift, Carlyle, Schopenhauer, Goethe, Nietzsche, Emerson, Thoreau, James, whose teachings tend toward the disintegration of the crowd-mind and emphasize the importance of self-analysis, were never popular in their own time, and the lip homage rendered them by posterity echoes hollowly against the walls of intellectual bondage.

## Tyranny of Crowd Spirit

Probably no modern nation has slid more readily into the channels of crowd-thinking than America. This may be because of the newness of the country, and the comparative sparsity and heterogeneity of the population, which might tend to draw people into groups and to make them think as groups. It is also probable that the unparalleled abundance of opportunities which have attracted people to this country has so sharpened the quest for material advantages, with the resultant rivalries and suspicions, that the capacity for objective self-analysis has been woefully neglected.

A not unfriendly critic, de Tocqueville, the Frenchman, who visited America in 1830, noted the whole trend toward impulsive crowd-action, which he called the "tyranny of the majority." While he praised whatever appeared meritorious to him, he was equally free in reporting our shortcomings. Much of his comment is so applicable today, that the following few paragraphs will bear quoting, and we may yet profit by the frank criticism of this observant visitor:

"America is therefore a country in which, lest anybody be hurt by your remarks, you are not allowed to speak freely of private individuals, of the State, or the citizens, or the authorities, of public or private undertakings, in short of anything at all, except perhaps the climate and the soil, and even then, Americans will be found ready to defend both as if they had concurred in producing them.

"The American submits without a murmur to the authority of the pettiest magistrate. This truth prevails even in the trivial details of national life. . . . If an American were condemned to confine himself to his own affairs, he would be robbed of one-half of his existence; his wretchedness would be unbearable.

"The French under the old régime held it for a maxim that the King could do no wrong. The American entertains the same opinion with regard to the majority. . . . The majority, therefore, in that country exercises a prodigious actual authority and a power of opinion which is nearly as great (as that of the absolute autocrat). No obstacles exist which can impair or even retard its progress so as to make it heed the complaints of those whom it crushes upon its path. This state of things is harmful in itself and dangerous for the future.

"I am not so much alarmed by the excessive liberty which reigns in that country as by the inadequate securities which one finds against tyranny. When an individual or party is wronged in the United States, to whom can he apply for redress?

"It is in the examination of the exercise of thought in the United States that we clearly perceive how far the power of the majority surpasses all the powers with which we are acquainted in Europe. At the present time the most absolute monarchs in Europe cannot prevent certain opinions hostile to their authority from circulating in secret through their dominions and even in their courts. It is not so in America. So long as the majority is undecided, discussion is carried on, but as soon as its decision is announced, everyone is silent.

"I know of no country in which there is so little independence of mind and real freedom of discussion as in America. In America the majority raises formidable barriers around liberty of opinion. Within these barriers an author may write what he pleases, but woe to him if he goes beyond them."

If these strictures from a friendly critic seem severe, it is only because we are not given to analysing our own acts and motives. But aside from the severity, we should be concerned primarily with the question of the *accuracy* of the observations. The most superficial introspection of our national conscience will substantiate all that has been said.

### Crowd Witch-Hunting

High and low, we have acquired a crowd-dictating and crowd-conforming psychology. Especially within the scope of the social sciences, the man who departs from the beaten path of orthodoxy receives little better consideration than did Friar Bacon or Galileo centuries ago.[2] The only difference is, it is not usually necessary to incarcerate him in a prison, because he can be as effectively silenced by separating him from his work and livelihood. No quality of intellectuality or moral principle, if non-conformist, is too rare to halt the onslaught of the witch-hunting crowd.

Eminent college professors have been turned out of their positions; clergymen have been forced from their pulpits; publicists have been driven from public life; writers and editors have been denied the medium of print; duly elected representatives have been ousted from their legislative seats; scientists and other professional workers have been harassed; lecturers and public speakers have been attacked and maltreated; men and women of independent mind have been ostracised in society; and numerous individuals not before the public eye have been persecuted in countless ways. This coercion, covering all the above outrages and many that are not here mentioned, was exercised, not for committing any crime or misdemeanor whatever, but merely for having and

[2] "There never was a liberal idea which has not been unpopular; never an act of justice which has not caused scandal; never a great man who has not been pelted with potatoes or struck by knives. The history of human intellect is the history of human stupidity, as M. de Voltaire said.''—G. Flaubert, *Lettres à Georges Sand*.

*expressing* an opinion that did not bear the approved imprint of the crowd.

The tendency toward hysterical conformist legislation, which seeks to make people act and even *think* alike, has been noted. Not only morals and social conduct must be regulated by legislative reform waves, but personal habits and tastes as well. Everything done in crowd-fashion is popular with the majority. Its effectiveness is considered synonymous with righteousness and success. From industrialism to religion the popular ideal is epitomized in mass, jazz and conformity. Ford production and Billy Sunday evangelism are the supreme achievements in their respective fields.

The crowd-impulse to act and hunt in packs is so manifold in its expression that it may be called the psychopathology of every-day life. It offers one of the best means of observing the Caveman at work. Rational, directed thought, consideration of and regard for consequences, are quite foreign to its method. A realization of its mechanism enables us to understand the prevalence of riots, lynchings and other mob activities. Instead of expressing our amazement over the occurrence of these shocking affairs, we can see that they are the grosser evidences of phenomena that are taking place about us every day. Almost any aggregation of people will furnish the mob-spirit, and it requires only the immediate incentive (or excuse), and some sensation-seeking individual or medium, to set off the explosive energy that lies underneath the skins of the crowd.  As Mr. Martin says, "A crowd is a device for indulging ourselves in a kind of temporary insanity by all going crazy together."

## Race Riots and Pogroms

The race riot at Tulsa, Oklahoma, in the Spring of 1921, illustrates this example of grim realism better than any other recent occurrence.  Within an unbelievably short space of time, and from the most insignificant apparent cause, a conflagration was under way which resulted in the loss of scores of lives and millions of dollars  worth of property.

The rôle played in this catastrophic event by a sensational newspaper is a crushing indictment of the standard of journalism so largely prevalent. Yellow journalism is designed to cater to the explosive emotionalism of the modern Caveman, and its effect on him is frequently like a spray of oil on a furnace.

One editor stated that the horror was caused by "an impertinent negro, a hysterical girl and a yellow newspaper."  The riot—in reality it was a civil war while it lasted—started in the following way: A thoughtless, and possibly impertinent, negro boy stumbled as he entered the elevator of a hotel.  In an instinctive effort to regain his balance he caught hold of the arm of the girl who was operating the elevator.  The girl screamed.

A sensation-seeking newspaper reporter who happened to be near wrote a wholly false story of the negro's attempt to assault the girl.  The newspaper, seizing the story as a choice morsel for the gullible, and not attempting to verify the account, published it under scare headlines.  This was the tinder which set off the conflagration.   A white mob collected to lynch the negro, and a colored mob formed to defend his life.  All signs of constituted authority and "law and order" vanished, the mob spirit rose to unprecedented heights, and the conflict raged until the death toll ran up around one hundred and a considerable portion of the city was wiped out.  As by the wave of a magic wand, centuries of civilization were obliterated, the influences of religion and ethics were forgotten, and the primitive Caveman broke loose in all his old-time fury.

This horror does not stand alone.  Similar epidemics of slaughter have occurred within a recent period in East St. Louis, Washington, Omaha and Chicago, and homicidal outbreaks of less far-reaching consequences elsewhere.  When occurrences of this kind take place in far-away parts of the world, we attribute them to the fiendishness of inferior, barbarous people, whom we should like to "civilize" and uplift, and we sympathize profusely with the unfortunate victims.  So it is when we hear of massacres of the Armenians by the Turks, or of pogroms in Russia and Poland.

"Reforming" and "uplifting" are such interesting pastimes! As we know them, they are purely crowd manifestations, invariably associated with a "movement." They are interesting because they enable us to work on some other fellow—and so forget our own shortcomings. The puritanical group would reform all the rest of the people of the country and have them conform to its way of thinking. The people of the country generally would "civilize" and "Christianize" the Turk, the Chinaman, the Jap, the Hindu, the Zulu and the South Sea Islander.

Instead of beginning with the citizens of Tulsa, East St. Louis, Washington, Omaha, Chicago, and every other village, town, and city of the country, we speak of "Americanizing" the immigrant. We do not specify the particular standard, except in the most abstract and platitudinous terms.

Seth K. Humphrey reminds us in his book, *The Racial Prospect:* "And our boasted Americanism is not a cure for mental incompetency. The police blotters of our cities will show that the mobs which spring from nowhere at the slightest let-up of police control are mostly American-born, with scarcely an illiterate among them; yet they revert to the sway of their animal instincts quite as spontaneously as benighted Russians."

We might only question the use, or at least the meaning, of the term "illiterate" in the above statement. As a matter of fact, we know that illiteracy is rampant throughout the country. A great deal of it may not be elementary alphabet illiteracy, but there is a very pronounced degree of economic and social illiteracy, with all the spiritual and intellectual poverty and lack of insight that this implies.

## National Mobs and War

While the character of the mob spirit is a reversion to the Caveman and is latently present in every crowd, it is however usually local in its manifestation. A thousand different crowds in a thousand different sections of the country may surge with emotionalism over a thousand different incidents.

There is one paramount phenomenon—War— which not only unites all the scattered crowds into one national super-crowd, but it transforms every wheel of the social, economic and political mechanism into a means of furthering crowd-feeling and crowd-action. Not satisfied with all necessary defensive and offensive military measures and economic support, there is no end to the devices used to foster a pure and simple mob spirit on a national scale.

The atavistic desires that are repressed in normal times, cropping out only in mild and distorted forms through dreams at night, and phantasies, wit and other comparatively harmless ways by day, are suddenly released by war. Not only are the soldiers in the field vouchsafed a primitive outlet for pent-up emotions, but, as E. D. Martin says, "the whole nation becomes a homicidal crowd." It is looking for blood, and not only "the enemy within," but the ill-advised peace-maker and all others who express a thought or offer a suggestion that is not in tune with the prevailing martial notes, are flirting with the hazards of fate. If our neighbor's veneer of civilization is a little thicker than our own and he does not respond so readily to the primitive call of the tom-toms and blare of the war-spirit, we suspect his patriotism, or even call him traitor.

As Freud suggests, it is not that people sink very low in time of war; they were never so high in peace times as popularly supposed. Is there any other hypothesis to explain why men who, before war starts, are apparently humane and reasonable, will later give voice to the most violent and *lawless* outbursts against people who differ from them, and whose motives they may not understand? The fact that they hold a minority opinion is a sufficient indictment. "Hang them to the first lamp post," "Shoot them at sunrise," "Shoot them first and try them after," are the hectic suggestions offered by many citizens who have been brutalized by the spirit of Mars. The veneer has been rubbed off.

The passion that has been unloosed by war permeates every stitch of the social fabric. Rationality and lucid reasoning, so rare at any time, are scrapped with the arts of peace, and we are swept on every side by the turgid emotionalism of the day. We read it in editorials, fiction, poetry, news articles and all sorts of special write-ups. We hear it on the lecture platform, the vaudeville stage, in the pulpit, on the street, in schools, shops, offices and in our homes. It is constantly paraded before us, harangued about us; it flutters above us—is visible and audible everywhere.

In addition to the crowd psychology of war hysteria, there is undoubtedly a remnant of the parent fixation that contributes to the individual side of the emotionalism. There is a widespread identification of the country with the mother, and of the authority of the government with the father. The personification of a country is invariably a mother-image in patriotic drawings, as *Columbia, Britannia, la France;* although the governments are represented by father-images—"Uncle Sam," "John Bull", Johnny Crapaud.

Those who labor under the most inhibitions in times of peace are apt to be the quickest to throw off all reason and restraint when the emotionalism of the mob becomes epidemic. It is no uncommon thing at the fever heat of war to hear clergymen— the anointed spokesmen of the Prince of Peace— declaiming the dogma of the enemy's utter destruction, and the annihilation of all for which he stands. This is the tendency in all countries. However, as a clergyman's elementary urges are possibly more constantly repressed than the average, it is only natural, when the inhibitions of society are largely removed, that he should go as far as or even a little bit farther than the rest.

Romain Rolland, Andreas Latzko and other realistic writers have emphasized the emotional extremes of women during the World War. Their militant passion, as a rule, surpassed that of the men. As women normally are subjected to greater social restrictions than men, their reaction was more intense when the restraints were swept away.

One of the typical phases of war hysteria is the desire for suppression of inanimate things which are merely symbolic of the enemy. The speaking of his language is forbidden, likewise the circulation of his literature (even the classics). In preventing the singing and playing of his music, there is as much satisfaction felt as over a military victory. Anything suggestive of the enemy (no matter how commendable it may be in normal times) is taboo. Even favorite foods that have emanated from the culinary arts of the enemy are acceptable only after they undergo the chastening of being patriotically renamed.

This means that by banishing from the sight of our eyes and the sound of our ears all evidence of the enemy's existence, we feel the more secure and triumphant. Figuratively, we emulate the example of the ostrich and bury our head in the sands of self-delusion. By refusing to see any works or signs of the enemy, we unconsciously deny his existence. He is less of a menace to us.

Nothing so much excites the primitive, emotional nature of the individual, stimulates his endurance, and promotes his fighting qualities, as music—particularly martial music. Darwin observed that music has a wonderful power of recalling in a vague and indefinite manner strong emotions which have been felt by our ancestors in ages long gone by.

Throughout the whole of military history, music has played a vital rôle in martial combat. The conquering Romans charged the enemy to the accompaniment of trumpets and horns. A tradition tells us that the Hungarian troops are the worst in Europe until their bands start to play—then they are said to be the best. A famous Russian General stated that from the music the soldier absorbs a magic power of endurance, and forgets the sufferings and mortality. "It is a divine dynamite." Napoleon is accredited with saying that the weird and barbaric tunes of the Cossack regiments infuriated them to such rage that they wiped out the cream of his army.

Recognition of the fighting emotions of man requires that some substitute be offered for the utilization of this energy. It *will* express itself, either in a primitive way as a destructive, antisocial force, or it may be given an outlet along constructive, socially useful lines.

It should be obvious that an insight into the energetic constitution of man is a prime requirement for the ethical regeneration that is so ardently hoped for. The counsel of the early sage to "know thyself" is as timely today as it was nearly twenty-five hundred years ago. An insight into the mechanism of instinctive or automatic behavior will enable one to understand the belligerent feelings which well up from an ancient biological heritage. Most people know as little about this aspect of their organism as a Hottentot knows about the mechanism of an automobile. While myriads of unenlightened Hottentots are not attempting to run automobiles promiscuously in our midst, great masses of our fellow civilized beings are running about, absolutely uninitiated into the mysteries of the intricate human machine they are operating so blunderingly.

With a knowledge of the invisible mechanism, there will come some nearer approach to mastery in its operation—self-mastery. The ability to *control* emotions and *direct* energy will be acquired only when some idea of the processes of these forces is generally known. It will be noted that I have not suggested to "suppress" emotions. I have emphasized "control," and *control* is a form of *expression*.

Prominent among the constructive and socially desirable forms of emotional outlet are athletics, sports and other healthy rivalries. And in addition to physical endeavor, emotional expression is afforded in the arts and crafts, in dancing, in song, in love, in *life*. There is a wide field of social welfare work that can utilize all the spiritual forces available. Barren moralizing may easily be dispensed with. The recognition of a present-day application of these forces is in contrast to the old-fashioned religious code which focused its attention on, and idealized, the remote period of nineteen centuries back, and looked to the Hereafter for its reward. This left a spiritual gap in the present which can only be filled by a satisfactory means of expression. Constructive energy must be hitched up with some contemporary social force.

When all the primitive emotions are vouchsafed an outlet that is adequate to the ego-nature and serviceable to society, we shall be getting farther away from the dominant neurotic type that is so readily brutalized by the hysteria of war. Instead of demanding suppression and conformity, we may look for more worthy adversaries who shall declare, in the spirit of Voltaire to his enemy Helvetius: "I wholly disapprove of what you say —and will defend to the death your right to say it."

## BIBLIOGRAPHY

MARTIN, EVERETT DEAN, *The Behavior of Crowds*, New York, 1920.

LE BON, GUSTAVE, *The World in Revolt*, New York, 1921.

LE BON, GUSTAVE, *The Psychology of the Crowd*, London, 1916.

WHITE, W. A., *Thoughts of a Psychiatrist on the War and After*, New York, 1920.

FREUD, SIGMUND, *Reflections on War and Death*, New York, 1919.

RIBOT, TH., *Psychology of the Emotions*, New York.

DE TOCQUEVILLE, A., *Democracy in America*, Vol. I, New York, 1841.

# CHAPTER XIV

## THE CAVEMAN DISOWNED

The average good citizen may be safely permitted at large only because he keeps a few of his natural-born proclivities locked up.—SETH K. HUMPHREY, *The Racial Prospect.*

MANY of the nervous and physical disabilities, as well as mental aberrations, resulting from attempted suppression of the Caveman within, have been noted. There is, however, a distinct type of morbidness of mind that warrants special consideration. This refers to the crusading puritan, the professional reformer, and the self-appointed guardian of other people's morals.

If this group of the population is small in numbers, the numerical handicap is amply compensated for by great activity and lustiness of voice. It is forever in action, and always heard. Morever, because of the indiscriminate crowd-impulsiveness of the people, described in the preceding chapter, it is remarkably effective in accomplishing its superficial and frequently negative aims—the enactment of repressive Blue Laws, for instance. The fact that it makes a "moral" issue out of its undertakings gives them a touch of sanctity, which often places at a disadvantage those who question their wisdom, propriety or rationality.

The particular mental kink that is responsible for this phenomenon, which in its extremes is nothing less than a psychopathological condition, is a deep, burning obsession—in substance, a genuine neurosis.

The operation of the law of compensation, physical and psychical, has been discussed. The neurotic puritan is essentially an example of this law in operation. The whole trend of his psychic processes is under the spell of an association of abnormal contrasts.

The individual who is always painfully good is likely to have the most vindictive disposition, which would have its primitive outlet in savage tyranny. He attempts to compensate for his anti-social propensities, constantly gnawing at his soul, by studiously assuming the personification of righteousness. All sorts of variations of this principle of contrasts may be noted.[1]

Cruel, extremely sadistic types, will characteristically affect acts of kindness and philanthropy. The late Monk Eastman, a notorious New York gangster, whose experiences covered a wide range of crime and degradation, was a fancier of pigeons —pets on whom he lavished much affection. The charitableness of thieves is commonly observed.

[1] Howard, the prison reformer, was a tyrant in his own house, and had a son who was insane. Nisbet emphasizes that piety is a frequent symptom of the epileptic condition.

## Puritanical Obsessions

The self-righteous person parades his virtue so diligently because, consciously or unconsciously, he is imbued with a feeling of sin, and in the desperate stress of self-protection, he throws his tendencies to evil in the opposite direction. This would be admirable if it spurred him to some constructive endeavor, which would strengthen his personality and develop his character. But, if he did this, he would cease to be obsessed by his inner conflict, and he would not longer need to display his goodness on dress parade. Always viewing the actions of others from a subjective angle, and applying to them his own motives, he believes them beset by the same temptations as he. So in trying to "save" others, by having them tread in his futile steps, he wastes his own possibilities and too often becomes a sanctimonious nonentity.

The inner struggle due to hatred of the "flesh" in himself, engenders within him a profound hatred of the flesh in others. Therefore, he does a vicarious penance for his own feeling of sinfulness by attempting to punish the sins of others.

The man or woman who is distressed by every reference to, or suggestion of, sex in literature, in art, on the stage, or in certain costumes on the street, is emphasizing the subject above its normal importance. This self-consciousness indicates a pronounced degree of suppressed pornophilia—

love of the libidinous.  There is the mechanism of a perversion at work in the person who is constantly finding indecency in the actions of those about him.

There is the type of ultra-virtuous individual who glories in his own self-denial.  His repression of natural desires is carried to such extremes that there is a distinct pathological reaction.  Persons of this type may be compared to the "holy men" of the Middle Ages who subjected themselves to flagellation and other self-inflicted tortures of the "flesh" in order to demonstrate their purity of spirit.

As a matter of fact, it was their perversity of spirit that was hurting them, rather than the much abused flesh, which was simply behaving naturally, humanly, and therefore in accordance with the will of the Omnipotent.  Far from being the godly sort the canons and traditions have made them out to be, they were simply perverted victims of masochism.  The records of ascetics and ecstatics who flourished in the medieval period offer eloquent testimony of abnormalities due to repressions, with the consequent hallucinations, visions and trances that are so frequently manifested by the insane patient of today.

The victims of hyperæsthesia (over-sensitiveness to sexual stimuli) are particularly susceptible to puritanical fanaticism; or at least they are until they understand the unconscious motives that color their prejudices and dominate their actions.

An insight into the situation, of course, will tend to bring about a more rational and wholesome attitude. Confirmed neurotics of this type, however, get too much satisfaction out of their perverse state of mind to allow themselves an insight into their obsessions. In addition to the gratification they experience, the inner struggle causes them to fear peering too far into their own thoughts. They much prefer to project outwardly and see in others the disgust which they actually feel in themselves.

Even the hyperæsthetic subject who succumbs to his sensuality and becomes a profligate manifests this same trait. It has been universally noted that the Don Juan has the psychology of a prude, and is invariably found on the side that opposes a rational understanding of, and healthy attitude on, sexual questions. An above-board scientific discussion of sex is anathema to the libertine. The subject to him cannot have a normal, healthy aspect, because his type of mind identifies it with obscenity and filth, as does the hyperæsthetic who has not fallen publicly from grace. In the popular conception, they are morally as far apart as the poles, but psychologically, they are identical—obsessed by the same burning impulses, plagued by the same phobias.

The anæsthetic puritan, on the other hand, represents a radically different type of negativism. This designation implies frigidity, which in its true form is due to low sexual vitality or a constitutional organic defect (undeveloped genitals). Lacking normal sensation, persons of this type cannot understand the sexual interest shown by normal individuals, and are apt to consider them "low" and "vulgar."

Even the socialized phase of sex expression, as in art, literature, the drama, etc., does not interest them, because its appeal is lost on their erotically anæstheticised organism. However, they are usually tolerant. Devoid of strong desires and not obsessed by conflicts, they are not impelled to compensate for a feeling of guilt by pointing out a similar condition, real or imaginary, in others.

### Professional Reformers

That there is a difference between fostering in the community a more clean and wholesome atmosphere, with opportunities for healthy recreation, and subjecting the community to iron-bound repressions in order to satisfy the irrational and often perverted notions of self-appointed moralists, is quite obvious. The difference between these two aims is the difference between rational enlightenment and anachronistic fanaticism.

Making the community a more wholesome, healthy place to live in, morally and physically, implies more than spectacular outbursts against sensuality. It is strange that the typical "reformer," if he is really interested in improving the moral and physical condition of his fellow-man, so studiously overlooks the wretched housing and insanitation that exist in the slums and in many outlying country districts and industrial settlements, as well as other social and economic factors that are directly conducive to the disintegration of family life. The immorality traceable to adverse economic conditions can hardly be overestimated.

The professional reformer finds no opportunity for gratifying his inflated ego in facing the tremendous problems of economic and social consequence. The sensational vice crusader would find in the tedious rôle of constructive educational and social work no stimulation to his exaggerated, but repressed, sexuality. Hence, he follows a "calling" that furnishes him a morbid pleasure.

Reformers who describe in elaborate detail the iniquities they have investigated are always listened to with breathless interest. Billy Sunday's lectures for "men only" and "women only" were by far the most popular in the repertoire of that versatile evangelist.

The audience, fascinated by the revelations of wickedness and debauchery that are ordinarily proscribed in public speech, literally enjoy the unfolding of the tabooed theme. The listeners, in their engaging phantasies, are identifying themselves with the speaker who has plumbed the depths of some interesting "sin." The psychological reaction is exactly the same as with the readers of the latest sex-motive tragedy which is played up and profusely pictured in the sensational newspapers.

We are told of certain professional reformers who have large collections of obscene pictures, which are constantly being augmented, and which they exhibit occasionally to those they think sufficiently pure in mind not to be harmed.

The attempt to meet the problems of vice by the application of a non-sensational, scientific program, such as has been undertaken by various Social Hygiene organizations, represents the enlightened method, in contrast to the pathological activities of oversensual neurotics.

Modern puritanism is best exemplified in the person of the late Anthony ·Comstock, whose life history offers an interesting study from the viewpoint of psychopathology. His friend and biographer, Charles G. Trumbull, has unwittingly given many episodes in his book, *Anthony Comstock, Fighter,* which illustrate the morbidity of his subject.

Comstock's father was an aggressive, puritanical character, with the sadistic tendencies that run true to his type. The story is told that, to add refinement to his chastisement, he was accustomed to send young Anthony out to cut switches with ,which to be whipped for some juvenile offense.

As a youth, Comstock was a strong, husky lad, a vital type that would, with his training, have to undergo the struggle to suppress the healthy biological instincts of adolescence. Imbued with the puritanical conceptions of St. Paul, which were stressed in his early religious training, he lived over again the old conflicts between the Flesh and the Spirit. He conceived the instincts that tormented him, not as natural forces to be controlled and socialized, but as an unregenerate agency to be fought and obliterated.

Comstock, characteristic of the true zealot, believed himself to be operating under the direct supervision of God in his "fight against the Devil." Perhaps it was more than an unconscious association of himself with Christ when he wrote in the preface to his volume, *Frauds Exposed:* "I cannot expect to have better treatment than our blessed Master."

Armed with the assurance of his divine backing, neither the letter nor the spirit of mundane law was inviolable when it conflicted with the higher authority. One night in his youth, according to his biographer, he "went up to the gin-mill, wrenched off a shutter, climbed in, opened the faucets and drained off on to the floor every drop of liquor in the place. . . ."

When he entered commercial life, after the war, "He had come to know young business men, over and over again, whose lives were plainly being ruined by their interest in the obscene pictures and literature and other devilish things they had access to. In his close contact with the young business men of the city, he saw them *falling about him like autumn leaves, withered by the blighting touch of the obscenities* that were the staple of so much commercialized traffic.''

How it must have exalted Anthony's feeling of righteousness to have been instrumental in saving some of these myriad frail specimens of masculinity from impending ruin in the lure of pornographic literature!

But the reign of censorship did not end with the onslaught on commercialized obscenity. Reputable art institutions and accredited medical and sociological publications were also visited by the uninvited wrath of the indefatigable crusader.

Mr. Comstock went as far as to bring into court the clerk in the office of the Art Students' League who was giving out a prospectus of his institution containing reproductions of specimen drawings from the nude that had been made by students in the League's life class.

In 1916, the professional puritans of New York succeeded for several months in preventing the public sale, on the grounds of obscenity, of *The Sexual Question* by Dr. August Forel. This work has been recommended by physicians and educators the world over as one of the most able and wholesome expositions of sex problems ever written. Dr. C. W. Saleeby, the eminent authority on eugenics, says of it in his *Parenthood and Race Culture:* ''If the reader desires the name of only one book, that is certainly *The Sexual Question,* by Professor August Forel. This has no rival anywhere and cannot be overpraised.''

But the neurotic censors of our public morals thought differently, and it was only when, in the face of a wide discussion of the merit of the work, they became in danger of public ridicule, that the ban was quietly withdrawn. In this, as in many instances, it was a recurrence of the old struggle between science (knowledge) and fanaticism (ignorance), the latter posing as a moral savior.

### Blanket Social Inhibitions

On the purely sexual phase of the subject, it should be apparent to all that sex truths are infinitely more desirable than sex lies, which are bound to creep in if the truth is barred out. But the fact is the term ''sex,'' and everything associated with it, so unbalances the neurotic puritan that he cannot seem to discriminate between the clean and wholesome on the one hand, and the perverted and degraded on the other.

The idea of putting this type of person in a position of authority over matters that affect the lives, health and happiness of the people would be grotesque if it were not so tragic. It is like permitting engineers who can not distinguish between danger and safety signals to run railroad trains.

Sex, too, has its danger and safety signals, but

the sexually color-blind fanatics are unable to distinguish one from the other.

In commenting on the blanket inhibitions of organized puritanism by attempting to control private life through the police power and other repressive means, Professor Franklin H. Giddings offers the following incisive remarks:[2]

". . . It will attempt to prohibit many amusements that are in no sense public nuisances and to oversee others, to censor books, plays, newspapers and works of art, to dictate medical prescriptions, to inspect and measure the clothing of women, to prohibit tobacco as it has prohibited wine, and to say how adults may and may not spend their time on Sunday. This program makes a strong appeal to fanatics, to morons unable to pass the Alpha intelligence test who throng revival meetings, and above all, to the hosts (that Michael and Gabriel working in shifts could not number) of men and women incompetent to earn a decent living in the competent professions for whom the enterprise of making people good by law provides salaries at the expense of taxpayers."

Even a superficial understanding of the crusading puritan and professional reformer reveals the pleasure-motive as the goal of his satisfaction. All aggressive persons of this general type are pronouncedly sadistic in their psychological make-

[2] From "Can the Church Be Saved?" *The Independent*, August 20, 1921.

up, and no small part of their satisfaction is. in
the exhilarating feeling they experience over the
punishment of their victims. The elimination of
the evil, real or fancied, is actually secondary to
the infliction of the punishment.

In considering these characteristics, we recur
to an early prototype, Tertullian, one of the
Church Fathers, who is said to have declared that
one of the principal pleasures of the saints in
heaven is to gaze over the battlements at sinners
suffering in the flames of hell below.

The puritanical type of mind is notoriously
innocent of constructive qualities. All its frequently remarkable energy is devoted to repression and suppression, without much sense of discrimination between the helpful and the harmful.
The negative impulsiveness, or lack of coördination with reality, is the hallmark of the neurotic.

The puritan feels within himself the sway of
the elemental urges. Not understanding them,
and feeling them to be in conflict with his ethics
and ideals, he fights and struggles to overcome
them. The negativism of his life is the result of
this psychological conflict. Instead of accepting
his biological heritage, and adapting it to the requirements of social life, he blindly attempts to
deny his primitive personality: *the Caveman is
disowned*. But he nevertheless exists, and behaves
the worse for the irreconcilable treatment ac-
corded him.

## BIBLIOGRAPHY

SCHROEDER, THEODORE, *Free Press Anthology*, New York, 1909.

MENCKEN, H. L., *A Book of Prefaces*, New York, 1919.

COMSTOCK, ANTHONY, *Frauds Exposed*, New York, 1880.

TRUMBULL, C. G., *Anthony Comstock, Fighter*, New York, 1913.

SCHROEDER, THEODORE, *Obscene Literature and Constitutional Law*, New York, 1911.

RINALDO, JOEL, *Psychoanalysis of the Reformer*, New York, 1921.

# CHAPTER XV

## THE CAVEMAN AND THE GENIUS

*Men of genius summarize in a single type many separate personalities, and bring new persons to consciousness in the human race.—GUSTAVE FLAUBERT.*

THERE is a common tendency to accept genius as the acme of human perfection. This conception is largely due to the indiscriminate lauding of "great men" in biographical and historical works. Their wonderful achievements are pointed out, in some cases exaggerated, and their weaknesses and shortcomings are often ignored, or concealed in a gloss of romance. Besides, time tends to smooth over the rough edges of character, and obscure the faults of personality, leaving only the outstanding accomplishments to be observed and admired. And as most geniuses achieve a full measure of recognition long after they are dead, the memories which survive are centered upon their supreme attainments rather than upon their personalities.

A critical review of the lives of the world's greatest geniuses, however, demonstrates that their marvellous capacities for achievement were often balanced by character weaknesses and neuropathic traits of proportional magnitude.

These luminous individuals had developed their intellectual or emotional powers to an extraordinary degree, but they had not overcome, or eliminated, the Caveman within themselves. Not only had he not been eliminated, but he was ever asserting himself, as positively as in the most ordinary man on the street, and much more effectively.

The meteor of genius runs the gamut of all the psychoses, neuroses, hysterias, obsessions, hallucinations, epilepsies, and other derangements. Forms of insanity are by no means uncommon. All of these manifestations are evidences of the Caveman coming in contact with the restrictions of his environment. It is a conflict between the primitive, elemental urges and the requirements of society—some necessary and constructive, others ridiculous and even destructive.

There has been wide speculation as to the nature and cause of genius. Locke, Helvetius and other early authorities ascribed all intellectual superiority to education. A later group, under the influence of Galton, has given all credit to heredity. Schopenhauer makes the statement that "genius is simply the completest *objectivity;* i.e., the objective tendency of the mind, as opposed to the subjective, which is directed to one's own self."

Genius, according to Goethe, is only related to its time by its defects. Oliver Wendell Holmes conceived genius to be a "creating and informing spirit which is with us and not of us.'' Dr. Johnson maintained that genius resulted from a mind of large general powers being turned in a particular direction.

A number of distinguished thinkers, notably Lombroso, have insisted that genius is closely allied to insanity, and the famous Italian psychiatrist gives a vast amount of evidence in substantiation of this claim.

Other competent observers have asserted that genius is a condition far removed from mental disorder. Charles Lamb, overlooking the fact that he himself had been confined in an asylum, stated: ''The greatest wits (or genius in the modern sense) will be found to be the sanest writers.''

Herbert Spencer regarded the great man as the product of many coördinated social influences over which he personally has no control. Nisbet accepts a similar view, tinged with a degree of mechanistic fatalism, maintaining that genius is essentially a manifestation of nerve energy, and that the scope of a man's faculties is necessarily determined by a physical organization over which he has no control.

William James, with his characteristic originality, offered this view: ''The causes of production of great men lie in a sphere wholly inaccessible to the social philosopher. He must accept geniuses as data, just as Darwin accepts his spontaneous variations. For him, as for Darwin, the only problem is: How does the environment affect

them, and how do they affect the environment?
Now, I affirm that the relation of the visible environment to the great man is in the main exactly
what it is to the 'variation' in the Darwinian
philosophy. It chiefly adopts or rejects, preserves
or distorts—in short selects him.''

### Artistic Genius

All of these ideas of genius are interesting, some
really enlightening. But, after all, it is not so
much opinions we are after as the evidence to
form our own conclusions regarding the two-sided
character of genius—the creative, social side, and
the primitive, unadaptive side.

Space will not permit giving even the most cur-
sory résumé of all the material that is available
in this connection. It will therefore be possible
to consider only the more notable characters in
the history of art, literature, philosophy, statesmanship, science and religion, and to allude to
some of the pathological evidences.

The family correspondence of Michel Angelo
shows him to have been of a suspicious, irritable
nature, wanting in calm judgment, which led to
continuous trouble to himself and his friends.
Nothing but a morbid condition of mind could
explain his violent letters and frequent explosions
of temper. Some of his greatest works were produced while he was afflicted with severe nervous
ailments. At the age of fifty-six he is described

as suffering from sleeplessness, weak sight, pains in the head and giddiness. In 1544, when the artist was ill in Rome, he wrote to his nephew, who hastened to his bedside: "You are come to kill me, and to see what I leave behind. . . ." He left a confession of his morbid melancholy in a letter to Sebastiano del Piombo: "Yesterday evening I was happy because I escaped from my mad and melancholy humor."

Biographical sketches of other old masters give facts from which significant inferences are to be drawn by the student of psycho- and neuro-pathology. Leonardo da Vinci suffered from paralysis, which incapacitated his right arm; Vandyck was melancholic, and died at forty-one of "disappointment"; Raphael, addicted to sexual excesses, died at thirty-seven; Rubens died of a nervous gout, which attacked him at fifty; Salvator Rosa degenerated into imbecility; Benvenuto Cellini had hallucinations of sight in the form of ecstatic visions; Giorgione, remarkable for his big body and big head, lived a wild life and was notorious for his erotic adventures.

Turner, the renowned landscape painter, who possessed a surpassing faculty for colour, had a mind whose general cast was little above the level of the idiot. Sir Joshua Reynolds, at the height of his fame, suffered a stroke of paralysis, and later felt a sudden decay of sight of his left eye, which resulted in total blindness of that eye. John Flaxman, the "father of English sculpture" in-

herited a rickety, misshapen body, which in early
years required the support of crutches. George
Morland, whose father and grandfather were also
painters, drew wonderfully at six years of age.
From the age of sixteen, he was a drunkard, a
spendthrift, and loafer, with the most vulgar
tastes. Fuseli, Lawrence, Liversege, Wilkie, Mac-
lise, Doré and Meissonier, also showed evidence
of pronounced nerve-disorder.

In the musical world, Beethoven displayed eccentricities which bordered upon insanity. He
was notoriously absent-minded and impractical.
From the age of thirty he gradually lost his hearing, and in his later years was completely deaf.
Mozart, who showed musical genius at the age of
four or five, inherited nervous troubles from both
parents. During the composition of the "Re-
quiem," he labored under the delusion that he was
being poisoned, frequently fainted and became
partially paralysed. In his thirty-sixth year, he
died of inflammation of the brain. Chopin during
the early years of his life was subject to a melancholy which went as far as insanity.

Mendelssohn suffered from epilepsy, had shiv-
ering fits and headaches, followed by periods of
unconsciousness. These disorders grew worse
until his death at the age of thirty-seven. Wagner
was a reckless and disorderly boy, infected
with the wildest mysticism. "The most striking
thing about Wagner," said one of his biographers,
"was the extraordinary energy that animated his

frail body, with its disproportionately large head and brow. Impatient, nervous, irritable, he seemed to take pleasure in rending in pieces men and things.''

Weber sank into melancholia and died of consumption at the age of forty-two. Schubert's constitution was worn out at thirty-one. Paganini, an inveterate gambler, was epileptic and consumptive. Schumann and Donizetti had nervous disorders which attained the proportions of insanity. Both became paralysed. Schumann was seized with suicidal impulses, while Donizetti, in his later years, was confined in a lunatic asylum. After a fit of savage anger, in which Donizetti had beaten his wife, he composed, sobbing, the celebrated air, *Tu che a Dio spiegasti l' ali,* which led Lombroso to observe, ''a remarkable instance of the double nature of personality in men of genius, and at the same time of their moral insensibility.''

### *Literary Genius*

Probably no major poet has had a more unhappy heritage of neurotic morbidity than Byron. ''Some curse,'' he wrote to a friend, ''hangs over me and mine.'' His father ''Mad Jack Byron'' led a dissolute life, and his mother was a woman of very unbalanced temperament. She even mocked her son as being ''a lame brat.'' Byron, as a child, feared this unnatural mother, and as a man he despised her. His life in Venice was marked by the grossest excesses and the keenest nervous suffering. Jeafferson, his biographer, informs us: "His harem on the Grand Canal to which he gathered frail women from the homes of artisans and the cabins of suburban peasants, was fruitful of scandals. . . . At night he would roll in agony through long assaults of acute dyspepsia, more often lie in melancholy moodiness and endure the torture of afflicting hallucinations. . . ."

So little is known of Shakespeare's life that it is quite impossible to obtain authentic information about his personality. Towards the close of the eighteenth century, Steevens gave the substance of a biography of the Bard of Avon in these words: "All that is known with any degree of certainty concerning Shakespeare is that he was born at Stratford-on-Avon, married, and had children there, went to London, where he became an actor, wrote poems and plays, returned to Stratford, made his will, died and was buried." Thomas Kenny (*Life and Genius of Shakespeare*), accepting the sonnets, in common with most English commentators, as pure autobiographical material, finds that they exhibit throughout a "teeming, unchecked, more or less disordered profusion of thought and imagery in the mind of the writer." Without any conception of the physiological influences on genius, Kenny concludes, from Shakespeare's unrivalled faculty of transporting himself into the state of mind of every character of human being, that the poet could not have possessed a very resolute character of his own.

Charles Lamb and his talented sister, Mary, were both subject to fits of insanity. Charles was confined for six weeks in a madhouse about his twentieth year—the period at which he wrote most of his sonnets.

William Blake, a contemporary of Charles Lamb, is a conspicuous example of the genius who dwells on the borderline of insanity. He had hallucinations of hearing—"celestial voices seemed to call to him." Later, hallucinations of sight beset him. He lived in the midst of historical figures of poets, heroes, and princes, which he took for reality. Moses, Homer, Virgil, Dante, and Milton were his constant companions in visions.

Swift's insanity was congenital. At Dublin University, he led a wild, nervous life, for which he was severely censured by the academic authorities. He suffered at various times from giddiness, deafness, impaired sight, muscle twitchings and paralysis of the muscles—all symptoms of brain disease.

Concerning Dr. Johnson, Boswell writes: "Johnson, who was blest with all the powers of genius and understanding, in a degree far above the ordinary state of human nature, was, at the same time, visited with a disorder so afflictive that they who know it by dire experience will not envy him his exalted endowments." The idea that he was on the road to insanity particularly obsessed him.

Cowper, a chronic sufferer, fell into melancholia at twenty-one. In his autobiography he says: "Day and night, I was upon the rack, lying down in horror and rising up in despair." He also described minutely his attempts at suicide—"the dark and hellish purpose of self-murder"—and how they were foiled.

Not long before Southey sank into imbecility, Carlyle wrote: "How has this man contrived, with such a nervous system, to keep alive for near sixty years? How has he not been torn to pieces long since under such furious pulling this way and that?"

Goldsmith lived the life of a ne'er-do-well. He was always in debt, notwithstanding that he received liberal support from his family. Referring to a continental tour, one writer stated that Goldsmith "disputed his way through Europe." He was corrected by a contemporary who said that he "begged his way through Europe." The nervous affliction from which he died displayed its most clearly defined symptom in a violent pain extending all over the fore part of his head.

Milton was subject to nervous disorders, of which his optic troubles and final blindness were manifestations. He lived most unhappily with his daughters, who found him harsh and tyrannical. He thought them undutiful and accused them of cheating him in money matters and stealing his books in order to sell them.

When Robert Burns said that poets have a "stronger imagination, more delicate sensibility and a more ungovernable set of passions" than other men, he spoke from experience. He died at thirty-seven, as an immediate result of drunkenness and exposure, but it is improbable that his irritable and nervous constitution, inherited from his father, predisposed to longevity.

Sir Walter Scott showed pathological symptoms from his infancy. Paralysis and apoplexy were the afflictions of his later years. Upon the death of Byron, he experienced an alarming hallucination, believing that he saw the image of his deceased friend.

As a child, Keats was violent and ungovernable, and manifested emotional extremes. During his short life—he died at twenty-five—this brilliant poet suffered much mental and physical anguish. His agitation, under the attacks of critics, is said by Shelley to have resembled insanity. His passions were so strong that he had to calm his nerves with laudanum.

Shelley was subject to pronounced hallucinations. At Eton, he was known as "Mad Shelley." Hogg writes that he had "singular caprices, unfounded frights, and dislikes, vain apprehensions and panic terrors."

"All biographies begin with genealogy," observed Bulwer Lytton, "and with reason, for many of the influences that sway the destiny that ends in the grave, are already formed before the mortal utters his first wail in the cradle.'' The truth of this statement was never more evident than in Lord Lytton's own case, as the eccentricities of both sides of his family were combined in him. In early manhood, Lytton's disposition took a morbid and even dangerous inclination. From the first days of his marriage, he mistreated his wife by biting, kicking and otherwise insulting her.

As a boy, Dickens was sickly and puny, and subject to attacks of violent spasms. He appeared to have outgrown this feebleness with early manhood, but as he advanced in years he became restless and irritable, suffering from gout and incipient paralysis. At fifty-eight he died from effusion of blood upon the brain.

In addition to these representative figures in the world of literature, space will permit only a brief comment on a few others. At school Balzac had an epileptic seizure. Flaubert suffered from epilepsy from his twenty-third year and his nervous attacks rendered him morose and unsociable during the remainder of his life. Alexander Dumas in his later years became an imbecile. Wilkie Collins was an acute sufferer from his nerves, which led him to form the laudanum habit. His head was misshapen. De Quincey, the opium-eater, was a' victim of general nervous irritability.

Heine became paralysed at forty-seven. Schiller passed through a melancholic period during which he was suspected of insanity. De Foe had an attack of apoplexy about his fiftieth year.

Henry Fielding's constitution was shattered by gout at forty, and he had a son paralysed. Dostoevsky was an epileptic, morbid and selfish. Tolstoy had hallucinations, and was in constant conflict with reality.

Fits of depression beset George Eliot in womanhood, and she complained of "terrible headaches." Eccentricity pervaded the Brontë family, which affected the three famous sisters, Charlotte, Emily and Anne. The neurotic proclivities of Edgar Allan Poe are well known. As a child, Coleridge was weak, self-absorbed, and morbidly imaginative. Thomas Chatterton, who has been considered the most precocious literary genius the world has ever known, committed suicide in his eighteenth year. Nathaniel Lee, whose compositions were praised by Addison, wrote poems and tragedies while confined in Bedlam.

### Political and Military Genius

There is a common impression that, whatever the defects of genius may be, they are confined pretty much exclusively to persons of artistic and literary faculty. As a matter of fact, no type of genius escapes its biological heritage. If it did it would cease to be human. And all genius, notwithstanding its great development in one or more directions, is basically human—sometimes "all too human."

From the earliest times of which we have record,

eccentricities of character and instability of temperament have been noted in great military commanders. Alexander the Great inherited his genius for leadership and no less his pathological nature. His father, Philip, had a violent temper and was addicted to drunkenness and debauchery; his mother, Olympias, was a dissolute, incorrigible woman, who, it is said, previous to his birth, had a vision of her son's greatness. Alexander died in his thirty-second year from sensual excesses. Perhaps he wept for other reasons than because there were no more worlds to conquer. Neuropathic symptoms are evidenced by an affection of the muscles of the neck, which forced him from birth to incline his head to one side. His brother, put to death by order of Olympias, was an idiot.

Julius Caesar, according to the authority of Suetonius, became subject to epileptic fits toward the close of his life. This is confirmed by Plutarch who states that Caesar fell into convulsions during the battle of Thapsus.

Pronounced nerve-disorders beset Napoleon Bonaparte, as well as his brothers and sisters. From boyhood, the little Corsican was irritable, morose, obstinate, domineering, and without trace of conscience. He suffered from habitual spasms of the right shoulder and of the lips. "My nerves are irritable," Taine quotes him as having said of himself, and the former adds, "the tension of accumulated impressions sometimes produced a physical convulsion." From the peculiar form and illegibility of his handwriting, Abbé Michon, the graphologist, maintained that Napoleon evidenced a morbid excitability of the motor centers, characteristic of insanity.

Wellington was decidedly an epileptic. During his career as a statesman, after the battle of Waterloo, his fainting fits were a subject of alarm to the nation.

The neuropathic taint of the Romanoff family clearly showed itself in Peter the Great. He was afflicted from infancy with nervous attacks which degenerated into epilepsy. His son, by Catherine, was similarly affected. One of these seizures is said to have held him stricken for three days.

Charles V, the greatest European sovereign of the sixteenth century, had a double heritage of insanity. He was a son of the insane Juana (who was kept in confinement for many years) and Archduke Philip, whose family also showed evidence of marked mental disorders. Charles stammered, was subject to melancholia, and showed strong scrofulous symptoms. His genius asserted itself in extraordinary mental power and intellectual versatility.

At the age of forty, Clive had conquered India and achieved a world-wide reputation and untold wealth. As far as book-learning is concerned, he was almost illiterate, but he was of the dominating type, and displayed marvellous capacity for leadership. Between his flights of emotional excitement and impetuosity, he suffered from depression of spirits, and committed suicide at forty-nine.

Frederick the Great combined the mad military proclivities and sadism of his father, Frederick William, with an intellectual vigor and passionate love of music and literature. His heartlessness could only be measured in terms of pathology—as Macaulay expressed it, "A nature to which the sight of human suffering and human degradation is an agreeable excitement."

The youth of Oliver Cromwell is said to have been given over to low, boisterous, dissolute ways, the truth of which is confirmed by his letters. He had a fiery temper, and strong neuropathic tendencies marked his conduct throughout life, as they did his whole family.

The well-rounded genius of Richelieu was manifested in ecclesiasticism, in statesmanship and in literature. Still, the Old Adam asserted himself in an epileptic state. Moreau informs us that on one occasion the Cardinal, in a fit, believed he was a horse, and neighed and jumped; afterwards he knew nothing of what had taken place.

No greater names are to be found in the annals of statesmanship than those of the Pitts, father and son. The elder Pitt, known as the Earl of Chatham, suffered from gout, which alternated with true mental aberration. Junius, in one of his early letters, referred to Chatham as a lunatic brandishing a crutch. According to Lord Mahon, he suffered "a dismal and complete eclipse of his powers for upward of a year."

William Pitt inherited his father's genius for administration and debate, together with the paternal gout. At twenty-five, he had not only risen to leadership in Parliament, but was Prime Minister. He was the victim of nervous disorders which culminated in the form of "flying gout," of which he died at forty-seven.

The greatest Victorian statesman, Benjamin Disraeli (Lord Beaconsfield) was subject to fits of giddiness, which he described as like a consciousness of the earth's rotation. Once he fell into a trance, from which he did not recover for a week.

That the sensitive soul of Lincoln was haunted constantly by the shadow of morbidity is not popularly known. His quaint humor and ready wit (unconscious attempts to compensate for the gloom that pervaded his consciousness) have taken the public eye from his soul-suffering, which, however, was indelibly impressed upon his countenance. On the day set for his wedding to Mary Todd, Lincoln did not present himself for the ceremony. He was found, near daybreak, wandering about. "Restless, gloomy, miserable, desperate, he seemed an object of pity." For days he was watched closely and all knives and razors were removed from his reach. He said, "I am the most miserable man living." Two years after the death of his first fiancée, Anne Rutledge, he told a member of the Legislature of his State that "although he seemed to enjoy life rapturously, yet when alone he never dared carry a pocket-knife."

### *Philosophic and Scientific Genius*

Not even the luminaries of philosophic and scientific genius, which assumes the highest development of the rational mind, have escaped the outbreaks of the Caveman. It is a long way back to Socrates, and the information we have concerning his temperament may be fragmentary, but there is corroboration of evidence which tends to prove that the father of philosophy was eccentric to an extreme degree. Many years ago, Lélut, the French physiologist, wrote a treatise proving that, on the testimony of his disciples, Socrates suffered, if not from insanity, at all events from sensorial hallucinations. He had long reveries or ecstatic fits; and he believed himself to be attended by a familiar spirit whose voice he heard.

To no single group is science more indebted than to the early astronomers, and yet nerve disorders afflicted these in some instances with disastrous results. Copernicus died of apoplexy, and before his death was "paralysed both in mind and body." Galileo, who finally became blind and totally deaf, was subject from his youth to chronic disorders accompanied by acute pains in his body, and loss of sleep and appetite. Tycho Brahe became weak-

minded in his later days, and died at forty-four.
Kepler was sickly as a child and died at sixty
of a violent fever accompanied by a brain disease
which baffled the skill of his physicians.

Newton suffered from mental aberration as his
actions, and correspondence with Pepys, Locke
and others, shows only too well. In explaining a
most unreasonable letter to Pepys, Millington says
of Newton: "He told me that he had written to
you a very odd letter at which he was much concerned, and that he had done it under the influence
of a distemper that seized his head, and kept him
awake for five nights together."

A maternal heritage of nerve-disorder manifested itself unmistakably in Bacon's life. A contemporary writer says of him: "His infirmity is
given out to be gout. . . . But in truth the general
opinion is that he hath so tender a constitution,
both in body and mind, that he will hardly be able
to undergo the burden of so much as his place
requires."

Giddiness and loss of memory attacked Faraday before his fiftieth year, although he lived to
the age of seventy-five. Cuvier died of a nervous
affliction, and his children of brain disease. Har-
vey, the discoverer of the circulation of the blood,
was gouty, violent tempered, and given to eccentricities.

Kant in his declining years became imbecile.
Descartes had hallucinations of hearing, believing

himself followed about by an invisible person, who entreated him to continue his researches.

In 1826, August Comte, founder of Positivism, fell into a state of insanity, and for nearly a year was confined in Esquirol's asylum. Two years later he published his *Cours de Philosophie Positive*, the "fruit of fourteen years' labor." He was vindictive in spirit and it is not known whether he ever forgave an injury.

Pascal, all his life a victim of extreme nervous suffering, was also subject to hallucinations, one of which was that there was a yawning abyss by his side. As a child he had a sort of hydrophobia, being unable to look upon water without falling into convulsions. Epileptic fits were the cause of his death.

John Stuart Mill was seized during the autumn of 1826, at the age of twenty, by an attack of insanity, which he himself could only describe in the following words of Coleridge's:

A grief without a pang, void, dark and drear,
A drowsy, stifled, unimpassioned grief,
Which finds no natural outlet or relief
In word, or sigh, or tear.

James Watt, the inventor, was physically an invalid. In his youth, he suffered agony from continued and violent headaches, which often affected his nervous system, and left him for days, even weeks, languid, depressed, and fanciful; at which times there was a roughness and asperity in his manner that softened with returning health.

In Jean Jacques Rousseau, we find a fertile mind that was plagued by a many-sided morbidity. He was in turn a hypochondriac, a melancholiac, and finally a maniac. One has only to read his *Confessions,* his *Dialogues,* and his *Reveries,* to gain an insight into the mental tortures of a mono-maniac. No longer able to put trust in any mortal, he turned like Pascal, to God, to whom he addressed a very tender and familiar letter; and in order to ensure the arrival of his letter at its destination, he placed it, together with the manuscript of the *Dialogues,* on the altar of Nôtre-Dame at Paris. Then, having found the railing closed, he suspected a conspiracy of Heaven against him.

Voltaire was hypochondriacal. "With respect to my body," he wrote, "it is moribund . . . I anticipate dropsy. There is no appearance of it, but you know that there is nothing so dry as a dropsical person. Diseases, more cruel than kings, are persecuting me. Doctors are only needed to finish me. . . ." His friend Grimm said he was even very angry when one dared to assure him that he was still full of strength and life.

Megalomania—delusions of grandeur—was not only the portion of Dante, Hugo, Heine, Balzac, Chopin, Bruno, and other celebrities, but Hegel, apparently was impressed with his own divinity. He began a lecture with these words: "I may say with Christ, that not only do I teach truth, but that I am myself truth.''

The statement of Lombroso that the most complete type of madness in genius is presented in Schopenhauer, may be too sweeping. Nevertheless, Schopenhauer's life represents some amazing incongruities of thought and deed. "From my youth," he writes, "I have always been melancholy." Like Rousseau, he was frightened by imaginary diseases. In Switzerland, the Alps aroused in him sadness rather than admiration. He was contradiction personified. He denounced women, and at the same time proved himself too warm an admirer of them. He preached sexual abstinence as a duty, but did not practise it himself. He was a great rebel in philosophy, although he had nothing but contempt for political revolutionaries; and bequeathed his fortune to men who had contributed to repress by arms the noble political aspirations of his countrymen in 1848.

The genius of Frederick Nietzsche, fired with an iconoclastic ardor, influenced by the pessimism of Schopenhauer, and aiming ever at a perfectionist goal, finally burnt itself out in the crucible of hopeless insanity. For a quarter of a century before his death in 1900, he suffered from excruciating headaches, induced by brain and eye affections.

"A man's genius is no sinecure," said Carlyle's wife, a most intelligent and cultivated woman. She spoke from bitter experience, as his irritability was excessive, and he treated her with gross inconsideration. In his diary, he gives us a glimpse of the turbulence within him in these words: "Nerves all inflamed and torn up, body and mind in a hag-ridden condition." For many years before his death his right hand was palsied.

Even such a constructive, scientific genius as Darwin was a victim of pronounced neuropathic symptoms. His will power and trained mind probably prevented outbursts that would have characterized a less methodical person. He had bad days when he suffered from "swimming in the head," or giddiness (frequently the equivalent of epilepsy). Like all neuropaths, he could bear neither heat nor cold. Half an hour of conversation beyond his habitual time was sufficient to cause insomnia and hinder his work on the following day. The difficulties in articulation of speech which he experienecd are also indications of a brain disorder or neurotic affection. Nervous afflictions also beset his father and grandfather, both men of extraordinary ability and versatility, and the noted Wedgwood family, one of whom was Charles Darwin's mother, and another (his cousin) became his wife.

Among the disorders mentioned in these pages, the frequent occurrence of gout will be noted. While popularly believed to be a result of high living, gout is known to be an important member of the various nerve disorders. Bouchard, a French authority, finds it intimately associated with insanity, epilepsy, hypochondria, asthma, St. Vitus's dance, etc. Suppressed gout may cause paralysis, hallucinations or attacks of mania. These troubles cease when the gout returns to the joints.

### Religious Genius

The prophetic visions of the founders of religions and sects, it need hardly be necessary to say, were ideas projected from their own unconscious mind. In boyhood, Mohammed had several epileptic seizures, the first occurring when he was four years of age. This caused great alarm to his nurse, who thought he was possessed by an evil spirit. His temperament was nervous and melancholic. More than once he attempted suicide and his friends were apprehensive over the state of his mind. Walking on the hill near Mecca one day, he heard "a voice from Heaven," and looking upwards he beheld Gabriel sitting with crossed legs upon a throne between Heaven and earth. The angel cried out to him, "O Mohammed, thou art in truth the messenger of God and I am Gabriel." After this, there came to him at frequent intervals the revelations set forth in the Koran.

Gautama Buddha, the *Enlightened One,* fasting under the sacred Bo tree, or tree of wisdom, fought out the inner struggle between desires and the will to renunciation. It is said that he remained fasting in this spot for "seven times seven nights and days, until the archangel Brahma came and ministered to him."

St. Paul presents an interesting psychological study, and all of his attitudes and expressions sustain the opinion that he was swayed by a strong neurotic temperament, which he designated as "a thorn in the flesh." His attitude toward women, which has so strongly influenced the Christian Church in this respect, is typical of the obsessional neurosis when it is bound up with a feminine phobia. His conversion was the result of a hallucinatory experience. As the enthusiastic leader of the younger Pharisees, he was among the fiercest persecutors of the Christians. Hearing that there was a certain number of disciples at Damascus, he demanded of the high priest a warrant for their arrest, and left Jerusalem in a disturbed state of mind. On approaching the plain of Damascus at noon he had a seizure, evidently of an epileptic nature, in which he fell to the ground unconscious. Soon thereafter he experienced a hallucination and saw Jesus himself, who said to him in Hebrew: "Saul, Saul, why persecutest me?" At Antioch he had a hallucination similar to that of Mohammed at a later period; he felt himself rapt into the third heaven, where he heard unspeakable words, which "it is not lawful for a man to utter."

Luther was subject to attacks of giddiness, and he has given accounts of hallucinations he had experienced. He attributed his physical pains and his dreams to the arts of the devil, but his descriptions of them give us a clear picture of nervous phenomena.

Ignatius Loyola, after a wound, turned his thoughts to religious subjects and, fearful of the Lutheran revolt, planned and founded the "Great Company" (the Jesuits). He believed that he received the personal assistance of the Virgin Mary in his projects, and heard heavenly voices encouraging him to persevere in them.

Hallucinations were the mainspring of the achievements of Joan of Arc. From the age of thirteen (significant as the climacteric period of puberty), supernatural voices and visions began to manifest themselves to her. She seldom heard voices without seeing a light, and when visited by the angels Gabriel, St. Catherine and Michael, she was *kissed* by these celestials and "felt they had a good *odor*."

Francis of Assisi, sensitive, æsthetic and loving, reacted to the mystic influences of his environment by having visions. On one occasion he thought he saw Jesus nailed to the cross, and felt the "passion of Christ impressed even upon his bowels, upon the marrow of his bones, so that he could not keep his thoughts fixed upon it without being overpowered with grief."

Under the influence of a vision, Savonarola believed himself, even from his youth, sent by Christ to redeem the country from corruption. One day, while speaking to a nun, it seemed to him that heaven suddenly opened; and he saw in a vision the calamities of the Church and heard a voice commanding him to announce them to the people.

In the midst of a religious revival, Joseph Smith sought divine guidance that he might know which of all the conflicting churches was the true Church of Christ. In answer to his prayer, the Father and the Son, two of the Holy Trinity, he contended, appeared to him in a vision, and forbade him to join any of the churches then existing. Directed by the angel, he found the "golden plates," containing a divine message to the faithful, and established in 1830 the Church of Jesus Christ of Latter-Day Saints, commonly known as Mormonism.

Swedenborg believed that he had spoken with the spirits of the various planets for whole days. John Bunyan, violent and passionate in boyhood, saw evil spirits in monstrous shapes, orgies of devils, archangels and what not. George Fox, the founder of Quakerism, experienced frequent visions, and every fantastic impulse that swayed him, he considered an inspiration from on high. Wickliffe was a victim of paralysis, from which he died.

In recounting these irrational and primitive manifestations experienced by some representative men and women of genius in various channels of activity, it should be needless to say that there is no intention to detract from or minimize their great achievements. Their works speak for themselves; and by their works they shall be known.

Nevertheless in anything approaching a well-balanced study of personality, it is necessary to consider *all types,* and the exceptional phenomenon of genius is one too rich in possibilities to be overlooked. We find that genius is a unique capacity for creative work in one or more fields of endeavor. It is a gift to which has been applied some positive measure of training or preparation, even if it is—as it proved to be in many cases—self-applied.

On the other hand, outside of the special realm in which the faculties excel, the genius is the same biological mechanism as the man in everyday life. The duality of his personality is even more marked than in the ordinary man. We are merely interested in proving that, in common with those less gifted, he has a dual personality. In too many instances his peaks of achievement are matched by inordinate short-comings. But the law of compensation is universal, and its application is more readily observed in the exceptions than in the commonplace. Where there are mountains, we must expect to find valleys.

### BIBLIOGRAPHY

ROYSE, N. K., *A Study of Genius,* New York, 1891.
GALTON, FRANCIS, *Hereditary Genius.*
HIRSCH, WILLIAM, *Genius and Degeneration,* New York, 1896.

SCHOPENHAUER, ARTHUR, *The World as Will and Idea.*
TURCK, HERMANN, *The Man of Genius*, London, 1914.
NISBET, J. F., *The Insanity of Genius*, New York, 1912.
LOMBROSO, CESARE, *The Man of Genius*, New York.
PARISH, EDMUND, *Hallucinations and Illusions*, A Study
    of the Fallacies of Perception, New York, 1898.
SCHWARZ, O. L., *General Types of Superior Men*, Boston, 1916.

CHAPTER XVI

## THE CAVEMAN SPLIT OFF

> There are—put it conservatively—two men in every man
> of us. How many women in one woman is quite another
> question. But that side of himself which a man presents
> to the world and that aspect of his character which may
> be discovered by a scrutiny of his solitary acts, are usually
> two very different things.—BEN AMES WILLIAMS, *Miching Mallecho.*

MEDICAL records afford a number of cases of individuals who have suffered from complete dissociation of personality for varying periods of duration. These well known cases of dual and multiple personality do not interest us here primarily as pathological studies, into which category they fall, but rather as highly exaggerated expressions of symptoms that are common in everyday life.

While the layman has long regarded cases of double and multiple personality as mysterious manifestations of the supernatural, and the older psychologists and scientists generally had considered them exceptions to the natural law, it remained for a newer, dynamic psychology to prove that they are a universal phenomenon. The abnormality is due not to the duality or multiplicity of the personality, but to the lack of coördination among its component parts.   In the words of Professor Boris Sidis : *"Multiple consciousness is not the exception, but the law.   For mind is synthesis of many systems, of many moments consciousness."*

All abnormalities, as a matter of fact, are "normal" traits highly magnified.   People who, for any one or more of many reasons, are unable to retain their decorum, or who lose voluntary control over certain of their actions, exhibit peculiarities that before had been held in check.   Their personality is *contributing* nothing *new*, but is bringing to the front material which before had been repressed out of consciousness or controlled in consciousness.

Dual personality, as a pathological state, is the result of a dissociation or "split off" of greater or lesser severity, and as a consequence of which the whole organism is thrown into confusion and chaos.   The Caveman, no longer submitting to even the pretense of intellectual control, breaks away from the rational moorings, and leads the primitive life he craves, until a reintegration of the psyche may be affected.

### Alternating Personalities

The case of Miss Christine L. Beauchamp is one of several that are best known in the records of neuropathology. This person, whose identity has been veiled in the pseudonym here used, was brought to Dr. Morton Prince in the spring of 1898. She was a young woman twenty-three years of age, a student in a New England College, and showed extreme "neurasthenic" symptoms, suffering from headaches, insomnia, bodily pains and chronic fatigue. These are very typical neurotic symptoms.

Failing to give relief by the usual methods of treatment, Dr. Prince resorted to hypnotism, which seemed efficacious, and the young woman was apparently recovering. Then there suddenly developed, while she was in the hypnotic state, a second personality.

The characteristics of the second personality, which called itself "Sally," were the very antithesis of the normal Miss Beauchamp. Sally was mischievous, gay, carefree, talkative, and denied identity with Miss Beauchamp, who was reserved and dignified.

Some time later, Sally asserted herself while Miss Beauchamp was in the waking state, without the influence of hypnosis, and thereafter frequently reappeared, alternating with the original personality. Sally's coming was always a source of trouble and embarrassment to Miss Beauchamp, on whom she used to play tricks and inflict all sorts of annoyances. She wrote her shocking letters, and on one occasion mailed to her other self a box full of spiders and snakes. When Miss

Beauchamp received and opened this package she fainted from fright.

Miss Beauchamp was devoutly religious, reticent, and most conventional. Sally was irreligious, disposed to flirt and fond of smoking cigarettes. Miss Beauchamp was nervous and tired easily. Sally was a bundle of energy, and among other distressing habits, she used to take long walks, and then permit Miss Beauchamp to regain consciousness, several miles from home, penniless and thoroughly fatigued.

Sally was full of the joy of living, recognized no responsibilities, preferred menial tasks to artistic or cultural pursuits; while Miss Beauchamp was depressed in spirits, well educated, and an accomplished musician and linguist. At one time, when Miss Beauchamp, in the despair of thinking she was losing her mind, attempted to commit suicide by gas, Sally, rising in the emergency, turned off the gas.

The case went from bad to worse, when suddenly a new personality appeared. This last personality remembered nothing that had occurred in Miss Beauchamp's life since 1893, although she possessed a full knowledge of her experiences before that time. The third personality, unlike Sally, was mentally developed, and, unlike Miss Beauchamp, was strong-willed, obstinate and sometimes deceitful.

Upon investigation, Dr. Prince learned that in 1893, Miss Beauchamp had suffered a severe shock, and that her illness began at that time. He was then puzzled to know whether this new personality was the actual Miss Beauchamp, and if the Miss Beauchamp he had known was not, like Sally, a secondary personality.

Realizing that only one personality could remain in control, Dr. Prince sought to bring the matter to a head. Rather by accident, he discovered that, under hypnotism, the primary personality and the newest personality merged into one. This suggested to him the possibility of achieving his end by the fusion of the three personalities into one well-rounded entity.

Again there was unexpected trouble, because, when released from the hypnotic state, the two personalities disintegrated, so that either the latest or the original personality assumed erratic control. Finally, after months' more treatment, and all of seven years from the time the case come under his observation, Dr. Prince found that he had to match wits with Sally, who had all along frustrated his plans by causing the disintegration, in order to prevent the probable termination of her existence. Armed with this knowledge, however, Dr. Prince was at last able to bring about a permanent fusion of the personalities, as a result of which Miss Beauchamp developed into a normal, healthy woman.

*A Case of Complete Amnesia*

In the evening of April 15, 1897, the Rev. Thomas C. Hanna, while returning home in his carriage, alighted to adjust the harness and missed his step, falling headlong to the ground. His brother, after vainly trying to restore him to consciousness, removed him to the home of a friend and summoned medical aid.

When, after several hours, he regained consciousness, he was found to have suffered a total amnesia—loss of memory. All the sensory experiences of his twenty-four years were wiped away and his mind was as blank as that of a new-born baby.

He was a man of versatile capacities, and not only displayed intellectual ability, but had a mechanical turn of mind as well. He was known for his strong will and excellent self-control, and was more readily influenced by reason than by emotion. He was notably free from neurotic taint, and a number of his forebears were distinguished persons.

While his memory was a perfect blank, his intelligence had remained intact, as subsequent events proved. He was eager to learn, and remembered readily the things that were told to him, although everything had to be explained in the most elementary way. Once he had grasped the meaning of a word, he made no errors in pronunciation, used the tenses correctly, and in forming sentences combined the words in their proper order. His greatest difficulty was in the acquisition of the use of adjectives and abstract nouns.

The world was a chaos of sensations. He had no conception of objects, space or time. Even the simplest mental processes which gauge distance, form, size and magnitude, were totally lacking in perception. He did not know how to control his voluntary muscles, and, having no idea of the possibility of such control, he could not walk.

Although, as it was afterwards learned, the sensation of hunger was present in a great degree of intensity, he did not understand its meaning. When food was offered to him he did not comprehend its purpose, and when it was placed within his mouth, he did not know how to masticate and swallow it.

In the manner of an infant, he had to be taught the most primary acts of life, and he gradually learned to pronounce words by imitating definite articulate sounds and to grasp their meaning in association with certain objects. Characteristic of the early mental development of children, he used one word to indicate all objects having a point of common resemblance. The first word he learned was "apple," which meant to him food of all kinds.

The distinction between his own movements and the movements of others was puzzling to him. From involuntary, chance movements of his arms and legs, he learned the possibility of controlling his limbs.

This most extraordinary case was treated by Dr. Boris Sidis and Dr. S. P. Goodhart. Their great problem was not only to impart to him the common knowledge of a normal adult, but, if possible, to bring back the "lost" personality, of which the new personality had no knowledge whatever, and to synthesize them.

He was taken to the home of Dr. Goodhart in New York City, so as to have the most careful and constant attention. Seven weeks after the accident, about three o'clock in the morning, the original personality awoke and the Rev. Hanna found himself in these strange surroundings. He demanded explanations from his brother, who shared the room with him. All memory of his experiences intervening between seven o'clock in the evening of April 15 and the early morning of June 8, had vanished, and he insisted it was evening—the time of day when he lost consciousness.

About four o'clock in the afternoon of June 9, he fell asleep and when he awoke, his second personality held the field of consciousness, retaining all that he had been taught, but remembering nothing of the primary self.

With his growing knowledge, he soon gained an intelligent insight into his condition, but there were continual changes of personality, one alternating with the other. As in other cases of a similar nature, the ideals and tastes of one per-

sonality were quite the opposite of the other. The
Rev. Hanna was a rather austere, strait-laced
clergyman, while the secondary character enjoyed
burlesque shows, risque jokes and drank beer with
evident relish.

Finally, he seemed to be seized with an intense
inner conflict, as if the two personalities were
struggling for supremacy. He appeared helpless
to choose between them because they were both
of the same nature, and at the same time too dis-
similar to be fused.

"The struggle," he told his physicians, "was
not so much to choose one as to forget the other.
I was trying to find out which I might more easily
forget. It seemed impossible to forget one; both
tried to persist in consciousness. It seemed as if
each memory was stronger than my will, and still
I had to determine which I had to drive away.
Just before lunch yesterday, I chose the secondary
life; it was *strong and fresh,* and was able to persist. At that time the question arose whether I
could not possibly take both. I decided to accept
both lives as mine, a condition that could not be
worse than the uncertainty I was in. I then felt
that the oft-repeated struggle would ruin my
mind. . . . *I am sure both are mine.* They are
separate and I cannot fit the two well together.
Secondary and primary states have breaks and
intervals in them, as though there were periods
of sleep. *The secondary state is stronger and
brighter, but not more stable.*"

Gradually, with increasing insight, a sense of order was established in Hanna's mind, and the two erstwhile discordant personalities were brought into harmony. A compromise was effected between the over-sublimated, over-worked, over-repressed clergyman and the primitive, unadapted, uncivilized Caveman who for several months struggled to prevail.

### Boy and Girl Alternating Personalities

Until she was eighteen years of age, Alma Z had been in good health and was considered in every respect a normal girl. Then, as an alleged result of "overwork at school," she underwent a remarkable change. Up to that time she had been an educated, thoughtful, dignified, feminine type. With the change, she was transformed into a carefree, happy-go-lucky person, child-like in her attitude toward responsibilities, ungrammatical in speech, and with a limited vocabulary in keeping with her mental regression. Moreover, in contrast to the ill-health of the subject, the new personality was free from pains and aches, had a good appetite, and comparatively a good deal of strength.

The second personality knew the primary one and she called the former "Twoey" and designated the other as "No. 1." At first Twoey, who seemed to have the power of going and coming at will, would remain "out" for a few hours at a time, but later she prolonged her stay for several days. Then the original personality would return, with all the intelligence, patience and womanly qualities, so typical of Alma, but also with the weakness and suffering which characterized her illness. No 1 became acquainted with Twoey through descriptions given by those who associated with her.

According to Dr. Osgood Mason, who observed this case for ten years, there were some striking differences between it and the two cases we have just reviewed and others that come in the same general category. There was absent the friction between the personalities that is usually characteristic of these phenomena.

While No. 1 and No. 2 appeared to be in every respect separate and distinct personalities, there was a sense of continuity in the mental stream, as each took up the duties of life where the other had left off.

Furthermore, the two personalities showed their harmony of spirit by becoming fast friends. No. 1 became attached to Twoey because of the care and consideration she showed toward her, and for her good nature and wit, which was a source of amusement.

Twoey, on the other hand, respected No. 1 for her superior knowledge, her patience in bearing the burdens of her ailment, and for her commendable qualities generally. It was in recognition of these virtues that she took the place of No. 1 with pleasure to give her rest.

It is interesting to note that as Alma Z improved in health and strength, Twoey appeared less frequently, and her visits corresponded with conditions of fatigue, or nervousness and mental excitement.

In the course of time, Alma married and proved herself a good wife and an efficient housekeeper. The situation took a new turn, however, as Twoey reappeared one night, but only to announce that she was to vanish and that she would be succeeded by another personality, "The Boy." The newcomer attended to all the duties which devolved upon Alma, but was firm in declaring her male character.

Alma, the student, was familiar with Latin, philosophy and mathematics, and had committed to memory numerous poems by Browning, Tennyson, Scott and others. The Boy, on the contrary, was absolutely illiterate, although "he" displayed an intelligent interest in current affairs, and was particularly fond of musical and theatrical entertainments.

At a concert in the Metropolitan Opera House one evening, The Boy suddenly disappeared and Alma took "his" place for a short time. But she soon closed her eyes, and in the gradual transition assumed the more masculine countenance which characterized the personality of The Boy.

The same inner harmony prevailed with the addition of this new personality. The Boy knew Twoey and No. 1, and was fond of them both. Like Twoey, he expressed the utmost solicitude for Alma, and was anxious that she should recover her health and not need him any more.

## A Secondary Personality That Fled

Ansel Bourne, of Greene, Rhode Island, had in early life learned the carpenter trade. As a result of a sudden temporary loss of sight and hearing, in his thirtieth year, he had become converted from atheism to Christianity, and afterwards lived the life of an itinerant preacher. He had been subject to headaches and temporary fits of depression in spirits during the greater part of his life, and also had a few fits of unconsciousness lasting half an hour or less.

On January 17, 1887, Mr. Bourne, then sixty-one years of age, went to Providence and drew $551 from a bank. He paid some bills and entered a Pawtucket horse-car, with the intention of visiting his sister, and this was the last incident he remembered until his amnesia terminated several weeks later.

As he did not return home, his disappearance was noted in the papers and foul play was suspected. The police, who tried to trace him, sought his whereabouts in vain.

On the morning of March 14, however, at Norristown, Pennsylvania, a man who had made himself known as A. J. Brown, and had rented a small shop six weeks previously, woke up in a fright, and demanded where he was and how he came there. He said his name was Ansel Bourne, and that he knew nothing of Norristown, or of shop-keeping, and that the last thing he remembered— it seemed only yesterday—was drawing money from the bank in Providence and boarding a street car. The people of the house thought him insane, as did, at first Dr. Louis H. Read, who was called in to attend him.

However, upon telegraphing to Providence, confirmatory messages were received and shortly his nephew, a Mr. Andrew Harris, came, settled his affairs and took him home. Bourne was very weak, having lost apparently twenty pounds during his eight weeks' experience, and had such a horror of the idea of the candy store that he refused to enter it again.

It seems that about a fortnight after the disappearance of Mr. Bourne, this stranger arrived in Norristown, rented the store and stocked it with confectionery, fruit, stationery and notions. He carried on a small trade, and conducted himself in a very orderly, methodical manner.

Later, he was treated by Professor William James, who hypnotized the aged preacher and elicited from him a fairly connected account of his activities during the eight weeks of his disappearance. These details he was utterly unable to recall outside of the hypnotic state.

In the hypnosis, he said his name was Albert John Brown, that on January 17, 1887, he went from Providence to Pawtucket, in a horse-car, thence by train to Boston, and from there to New York, arriving at 9 P.M. and registering at the Grand Union Hotel, as A. J. Brown. He left on the following day and went to Newark, N. J., thence to Philadelphia, where he arrived in the evening and stayed for three or four days in a hotel near the depot. He thought of taking a store in a small town, and after looking around at several places, among them Germantown, he chose Norristown, about twenty miles from Philadelphia, where he started a little business of five-cent goods, confectionery, stationery, etc.

He stated that he was born in Newton, New Hampshire, July 8, 1826 (he was born in New York City, July 8, 1826), had passed through a great deal of trouble, losses of friends and property; loss of his wife was one trouble—she died in 1881; three children living, but everything was confused prior to his finding himself in the horse-car on the way to Pawtucket. He wanted to get away somewhere—he didn't know where—and have rest. He had six or seven hundred dollars with him when he went into the store. He lived very closely, boarded by himself, and did his own cooking. He went to church, and also to one prayer-meeting. At one of these meetings, he spoke about a boy who had kneeled down and prayed in the midst of the passengers on a steamboat from Albany to New York (an incident of which he was well aware in the Ansel Bourne personality).

The completeness of the dissociation in the hypnotic trance is evident when the subject said he had heard of Ansel Bourne, but "didn't know that he had ever met the man." When confronted with Mrs. Bourne, he said that he had "never seen the woman before."

In the secondary personality, induced by the hypnosis, he looked old, and his voice was low and weak. Altogether, he was a rather shrunken, dejected replica of Bourne. He complained of feeling "all hedged in" and that he "can't get out at either end."

A reintegration of Mr. Bourne's personality was never effected. Professor James summarized the case in this sentence. "Mr. Bourne's skull covers two distinct personalities." Two independent systems were formed within the mind of the patient. One belonged to his waking and one to his subconscious life. When one was removed, the other emerged.

Unlike the Rev. Hanna, for instance, he had a neuropathic family history, and he personally had a psychopathic and neuropathic disposition. His maternal grandfather seemed to have suffered from senile dementia. The early psychopathic attacks and melancholia of the patient have been noted.

## *A Case of Quintuple Personality*

The case of Doris Fischer,[1] reported by Dr. Walter Franklin Prince, is one of the most complex in the literature of this subject. It involves five distinct personalities. Doris was born of German parents in 1889. Her mother's family was of healthy stock, while her father's evidenced some strong neurotic traits. Her parents were well educated, but the father, on account of excessive alcoholic indulgence, was reduced in time from a responsible position to that of a common laborer, so that the family lived in poverty.

The mental dissociations of Doris were caused by three successive shocks, incurred respectively at the ages of three, seventeen and eighteen. The first shock is described as psycho-physical, the second psychical, and the third physical.

The father, a violent, sadistic type, caused the first shock when, in a fit of temper, he threw the little girl to the floor. Two secondary personalities resulted from this shock, "Sleeping Margaret" and "Margaret." The latter had no access to the mind of the former, and did not know that she existed.

Sleeping Margaret claimed that she spoke only when Margaret was asleep, and that she was use-

---

[1] "The Doris Case of Quintuple Personality," by Walter Franklin Prince. *The Journal of Abnormal Psychology,* 1916. Richard G. Badger, Boston, Pub.

ful warding off dangers mainly by influencing Margaret, and also at times causing "Real Doris" to hear or see that which she otherwise would not have perceived.

The subsequent history to the seventeenth year is gleaned from three sources, i.e., the memories of Real Doris, Margaret and Sleeping Margaret.

In her triple life from the age of three, one curious feature was that the primary personality was never the one to sleep at night. The moment she had reached the head of the stairs leading to her room, Margaret would come and continue, except for brief sleeping intervals, until she had reached the bottom of the stairs in the morning.

Margaret would do the school exercises for her until the studies became so far advanced that *she* was no longer capable, would write notes to Real Doris, play and "imagine," often for hours. In the morning, Real Doris would discover evidences of pretended banquets and other play. The primary personality was in control the greater part of the daytime, but there were frequent transitions, during which Margaret would play her characteristic pranks and make audacious remarks. In school, Margaret would come and perpetrate some antic or singular speech, and then go, leaving Real Doris to wonder at the laughter of the pupils and to bear the brunt of the teacher's reproof.

The fourth personality, "Sick Doris," as she became to be known, made her appearance with the death of Mrs. Fischer. Sick Doris, like the secondary personality of the Hanna case, was characterized by the absence of knowledge-content. Her intellect, however, was good and she readily learned. *Another personality,* Margaret, was her principal teacher.

Margaret taught her, speaking subliminally by the lips, and subliminally using the hands, alternating with Sick Doris. She pointed at objects and gave their names, and Sick Doris would then point and repeat the names. She performed acts and Sick Doris obediently copied them.

When she was eighteen years old, she fell heavily upon the back of her head. The new psychical entity which then appeared was designated as "Sleeping Real Doris," whose identity was strengthened by another fall some months later. The ambiguity of the names must not lead to confusion. Sleeping Real Doris was far from being Real Doris asleep; Sleeping Margaret had absolutely nothing in common with Margaret, asleep or awake. And Sick Doris was not Doris in a sick condition, but an entirely distinct personality.

When Dr. Walter F. Prince took the case under his care in January, 1911, the primary personality had not had a total of three days of continuous existence in five years. For the first three and a half years of that period, Real Doris had not talked with a human being a dozen times, and only three or four times during the remainder of the period, as she nearly always "came out" in her room, which had no view of the street.

In describing the change of personality from Sick Doris to Margaret, Dr. Prince states: "When the secret became known, and she was free to act out her true character (since the rule is that a secondary personality, in spite of its 'breaks,' endeavors to conceal itself from strangers), it was startling to see the stolid, mature face of S. D. dissolve into the laughing, mischievous countenance of a young tomboy. The very shape of the face altered, and her voice was strikingly different, strident at times, at others almost infantile, full of inflections and vocal coloring. . . . Alone of the group she was slangy, and she misspelled and mispronounced many a word of which the others were mistresses. She could not understand why R. D. and S. D. wanted to go to church —it was all '*dumm* stuff' to her."

As in all cases of alternating consciousness, it would be when the primary personality became weary that she "lost control of her synthesis" and a secondary personality took her place. The whole process seems to be regulated by the consumption of energy and consequent exhaustion.

Dr. Prince described in much detail how, under the continuous care of Mrs. Prince and himself (in whose home the patient lived for several years), the various secondary personalities of Doris gradually grew less pronounced—while the primary personality grew stronger. From a bewildering bundle of disintegrations, the personality of Doris Fischer was finally synthesized into a single entity, evidencing a high degree of nervous and mental health.

The striking feature of all these cases is the neurotic characteristic, highly magnified in these instances, of fleeing from a psychically intolerable reality. In all except the Doris case, the subjects were persons who had, through over-repression of the natural instincts on the one hand, and attempting the over-development of the cultural nature on the other, inflicted a psychic trauma or wound, the results of which we have reviewed.

It is significant that the two male cases, the best known in this field of study; were both ministers, and New Englanders, who have been most influenced by puritanical notions. Swisher, who writes sympathetically towards religion and the new psychology observes that clergymen are particularly liable to "breakdowns" on account of the severe repression which is a part of their education. "In fact," he states, "such repressions have often driven men into the ministry. Detractors have called the clergy the 'third sex,' implying a sexlessness among them."

Miss Beauchamp and Alma Z were young women who had attempted the ascent of cultural heights which grew intolerable to the primitive side of their nature—and the Cave-creature rebelled in a most dramatic way. The characteristics of all the secondary personalities were distaste for study or mental effort, disregard for conventional ideas and responsibility, and a childish, carefree attitude toward life in general. The fundamental requirements of nature, to a large extent denied by the mode of life of the subjects, were therefore obtained in a most abnormal way.

Doris Fischer, of a sensitive, impressionable disposition, received a shock at the early age of three years, which caused her to flee from the reality of her brutal father. She took refuge in inferior, much less sensitive personalities, which were not so susceptible to the harshness of her environment.

The primitive nature of every human being has its irreducible minimum, beyond which it will not and cannot be repressed or coerced. It must express itself, either in comparatively harmless and socially acceptable ways (which have been outlined in previous chapters), or, if denied these outlets, it will burst forth in individually destructive and socially objectionable manifestations. Nothing illustrates better the effects of over-repression and a one-sided expression of the energetic constitution, than these pathological studies in dual and multiple personality. They serve as a magnifying glass which enables us to see and understand many peculiarities, eccentricities and personal idiosyncrasies in everyday life.

## BIBLIOGRAPHY

SIDIS, BORIS and S. P. GOODHARD, *Multiple Personality*, New York, 1905.

PRINCE, MORTON, *Dissociations of a Personality*, New York, 1906.

PRINCE, WALTER FRANKLIN, "The Doris Case of Quintuple Personality," *The Journal of Abnormal Psychology*, Boston, 1916-1917.

BRUCE, H. ADDINGTON, *The Riddle of Personality*, New York, 1908.

TRIDON, ANDRÉ, *Psychoanalysis and Behavior*, Chapter III, New York, 1920.

STEVENSON, R. L., *Dr. Jekyll and Mr. Hyde*. Probably the most famous dual personality in fiction.

# CHAPTER XVII

## THE CAVEMAN PARTLY DISSOCIATED

*Doct:* You see, her eyes are open.
*Gent:* Aye, but their sense is shut.
—SHAKESPEARE, *Macbeth* (V. 1.)

THE cases of dual and multiple personality briefly sketched in the preceding chapter—which involve complete dissociation of consciousness—are valuable chiefly as highly magnified examples of commonplace manifestations. It is only with this thought in mind that abstracts of them have been included in this volume.

There is a direct relation between these uncommon expressions of the Caveman and the every-day variety. The difference between them is one of degree, and not of kind.

There are, however, intermediate cases, belonging neither in the extreme category of complete dissociation of consciousness for more or less extended periods, nor in the classification of "normal" attributes, such as dreaming, phantasying, etc. Nevertheless, in one form or another, they are common enough, and in the aggregate they loom large in the minor pathology of the day. Chief among these phenomena are stammering, somnambulism and epilepsy.

## *Stammering*

According to the findings of analytic psychology, stammering, in many cases, is due to a dissociation or split in the psychic stream. Like the forgetting of facts, well known to a person, it signifies a mental conflict. The conscious mind is desirous of giving utterance to something, but the unconscious mind, presumably because the words have an unpleasant connotation, attempts to withhold them. The result in one instance is "forgetting" what we had in mind to say; and in the other, the articulation is interrupted. There are, of course, some cases of stammering due to a defect in the vocal mechanism or the motor centers of articulation.

It has been observed that persons who stammer or suffer from an impediment of speech in conversation are often able to sing well, and sometimes even to deliver a lecture without stammering or any hesitancy in the use of words. This indicates that the trouble is psychic.

Nor is hesitancy of speech confined to stammerers alone. Every one, when a personal complex is touched, hesitates for a moment, until a compromise is reached with the rebellious factor in the Unconscious.

It is interesting to note, especially in recalling a foregoing chapter, *The Caveman and the Genius,* that stammering has frequently been observed in men of genius. Among them may be mentioned Aristotle, Æsop, Demosthenes, Alcibiades, Cato of Utica, Virgil, Manzoni, Desiderius, Erasmus, Malherbe, Charles Lamb, Turenne, Charles Darwin, also his grandfather, Erasmus, Moses Mendelssohn, Charles V, Romiti, Cardan, Tartaglia.

The story of Demosthenes' struggle, which resulted not only in his cure, but in his becoming the greatest orator of his time, is well known. His persistent efforts may have involved some factor conducive to self-analysis, however unaware he was of the process that actually aided him. It sometimes happens that a person, either by chance or diligent effort, gains an insight into the psychic operations, and thereby experiences a revolutionary change in adaptability, without really appreciating the nature and extent of the discovery.

### Somnambulism

Sleep-walking, or somnambulism, is very distinctly an example of split-personality. In a way it is quite analogous to the amnesia cases of the Ansel Bourne type. There are, of course, differences, mainly the comparatively short duration of the attack, and the fact that the somnambulist is actually in a dream state, even though he walks, while the secondary personality in amnesia may lead a life that is practically as complete as the primary personality.

Somnambulism is a dream *enacted,* as well as visualized. The normal function of the dreamer is that of a spectator watching the drama as it transpires. Always, of course, he is the object of central interest. The dreamer watches himself enact, either in a symbolized or an undisguised manner, rôles of life that appeal to his primitive self—his ego. In somnambulism, the process is carried a step further by adding mobility to the visualization. The drama may then become a comedy—or a tragedy.

In sleep-walking the dreamer's eyes may be either closed or open. If open, he does not "see" in the ordinary sense of the word, although impressions may be made on the retina which will influence his course. The characteristic precision of the somnambulist, which has led to the belief· that sight is employed, is due to the fact that the dreamer sees very clearly the material of his dream and he acts from the visualization. Accidents, therefore, are very liable to happen to the sleep-walker. When he talks he converses with the characters in the dream. If one speaks to him, he will ignore the remark, unless it is associated· with the utterance of a dream character. If this is the case, a conversation may be carried on between the dreamer and an observer.

Partial somnambulism is more common. This condition is present when the dreamer performs certain motions without leaving his bed. In a dream of ascending a hill, he may, for instance, work his legs as in the act of climbing. Movements of the arms, in emphasizing situations in dreams also are very common.

There is a most dramatic case of somnambulism cited which happened in a monastery. Late one night as the prior sat at his table writing, one of the monks entered the room. He paid no attention to his superior, but walked directly over to the prior's cot and plunged a knife into the bedding. Without a word, or any sign of recognition of the astounded prior, the monk calmly walked out of the room. The next morning, the monk told his superior that he had had a terrible nightmare. He dreamt that the prior had done him some grievous injury, and in retaliation he had gone to his room and stabbed him to death in bed. He said he experienced a sense of profound relief when he woke up and found that it was only a dream.

Sometimes incidents happen which are wrongly attributed to somnambulism. A person may awaken from sleep, arise and perform some task, in which he is deeply interested, and then return to sleep. Having forgotten all about the matter by morning, the individual believes he must have acted in his sleep.

Pierre Janet has set forth a number of interesting somnambulistic cases, among them being that of "Irene," aged twenty, who had for sixty nights watched by her mother who was dying of tuberculosis. The facts may be stated briefly as follows:

Irene had nursed her mother through a long illness which culminated in death. The circumstances connected with the death were particularly painful, and as a result the daughter suffered an intense shock. An abnormal mental condition developed, which expressed itself in symptoms similar to those of the ordinary somnambulist. Whenever an attack occurred, Irene, regardless of what she was doing, housework or what not, would suddenly cease her occupation, and proceed to live over again the pathetic scene at her mother's deathbed with all the realism of an accomplished actress. While thus engaged, Irene was absolutely unconscious of anything that transpired in her environment. She heard nothing that was said to her, and saw nothing but the phantom scene in which she was living at the moment.

The drama would end as abruptly as it had begun, and Irene would then return to her occupation where she had left off, without being aware of the fact that it had been interrupted. After the lapse of several days, she would experience another somnambulism like the first in every detail, starting and ending in the same sudden manner. When interrogated during the apparently normal intervals, it would be found that no recollection of the somnambulistic experience remained. Further, she had lost all memory of her mother's illness and death. She talked about her mother in the most matter of fact way, and was rebuked by her family for her cold indifference to the subject.

The relation between the complex and the pathological symptoms is very clear in this case. The memory of the mother's illness and death was extremely painful and distressing to Irene. As a result, there arose a conflict in her mind between the system of ideas connected with the misfortune and her personality as a whole. In struggling to overcome this conflict, the mechanism of repression was resorted to, and the painful complex became detached from the remainder of the mind. Thus were banished from consciousness all memories of the tragic event. But, while beyond the realm of consciousness, the memories were not destroyed, consequently they returned with all their old emotional stress and tension, in a somnambulism.

### Partial Amnesia

The phenomenon of partial amnesia is as interesting to observe as complete loss of memory. The Irene case represents partial amnesia (having forgotten the fact of her mother's sickness and death), combined with the somnambulistic feature.

Bousfield relates the case of a patient who had

completely forgotten how his two intimate friends had come to their death, although he was standing near them at the time and saw the shell explode which killed them both. One of his friends had the whole back of his head blown away, and the other his abdomen ripped open. The horrible event was completely repressed from conscious memory, *as well as associations connected with the event which might have led to its remembrance.* A complete small section of his life was "split off from consciousness" and forgotten. A cure was affected as the memories were gradually revived by the method of free association practised in psychoanalysis.

Shell shock, in fact, is a form of psychoneurosis, which appears to be a compensation for the repressed self-protection urge. Hysterical blindness or deafness is a means of protection from terrifying sights and sounds; aphasias and abnormal gait necessitate the man's removal from the field of danger; and regression to infantile levels relieves him of the responsibilities of adulthood and assures him safety as a non-combatant.

Bram considers the term shell shock a misnomer and a term misleading in its implications. He emphasizes the similarity between the symptoms of shell shock and exophthalmic goitre, and believes that the great majority of shell shock patients are subjects of either an aberrant or a true form of Graves' disease.

We are told that goitre, associated with cardiac

and nervous manifestations, has been a problem in armies of the past. "Graves' disease is a chronic condition of 'fright, fight and flight,' as evidenced by the typical picture of perpetual terror in the well-developed case (bulging eyes, anxious expression, and trembling of the body)." These are definite symptoms of endocrine disturbances, particularly of the adrenals and thyroid glands.

There are some amnesia cases well known in the history of medicine, on which analytic psychology throws a new and significant light. Abercromby relates that a surgeon, whose head was injured by a fall from his horse, could give instructions for treating his wound, but completely forgot the existence of his wife and family for three days.

Forbes Winslow tells of a young married woman who, after a period of debility, lost all sense of the time that had elapsed since the day of her marriage. She remembered with remarkable vividness every previous event of her life; but when her husband approached her she repudiated all knowledge of or relation to him. She acted in the same way with regard to her child. Her parents and friends by their influence succeeded in persuading her that she was in reality married and had given birth to a son, but she beheld her child without being able to imagine how she had come by him.

After an attack of apoplexy a patient of Brown-

Sequard's lost all memory of events that had occurred during a period of five years. This period, which comprised his marriage, finished about six months before the attack. As a result of a blow on the head a man is said to have forgotten his Greek, but nothing else.

The difficulty that students have in wrestling with Greek is proverbial. What is more probable than that the man last mentioned had, in the drudgery of his early study of Greek, formed a positive antipathy toward the subject. Nevertheless, by force of will he had overcome this intellectual revulsion; but when his will power had become somewhat impaired from the blow on the head, he took the line of least resistance and "forgot" those memories which were distasteful to him.

All the other cases are concerned with domestic relations. And it is significant that in each instance the patient had lost all "memory" either of the existence of the conjugal partner and the family, or of everything happening during the period of married life. As marriage always represents a profound change in one's life, and involves added responsibilities and cares which are not attractive to the purely egotistical side of human nature, what is more natural than that in a crisis, when rational judgment is vitiated, the personality should symbolically revert to the more care-free life of the unmarried state. That there is no *consciousness* of this motive means nothing, as we know from the several cases which have been reviewed in some detail. With a reversion to a childhood mental level, due to an accident or other misfortune, there is the unconscious desire to enjoy the child's freedom from adult responsibilities.

### Epilepsy

The completeness of psychic dissociation in epilepsy, of course, depends upon the severity of the fit. The nature of the attacks varies from hysteria-like symptoms to manifestations resembling certain psychoses. It has been observed that epileptics are unusually sensitive beings, whose submissiveness readily gives way to the most extreme exhibitions of rage, culminating in a paroxysm. The frequency of epilepsy in men of genius, which has been noted, indicates the affinity of this affliction to sensitive, high-strung natures.

At the age of seventeen, Dostoevsky wrote to his brother Michael, "There is no way out of my difficulties. I have a plan. I am going to become insane." He did, indeed, become an epileptic. It is probable that the ecstatic experiences in his fits were a redeeming psychological compensation for the misery he endured in his "normal" state.

"I always awaited with impatience," said a patient of Francis Willis (*A Treatise on Mental Derangement*), "the accession of the paroxysms of insanity, since I enjoyed during their presence a high degree of pleasure. . . . Everything appeared easy to me. No obstacles presented themselves in theory or in practice.''

Among negative, inferior types, epileptic seizures seem to present themselves when the individual is unable to meet a certain situation, which a stronger character would strive to master. Submitting to the attack is a means of retreating from the harsh demands of reality, and at the same time it gives the victim an apparent advantage. It satisfies the unconscious ego-craving in this respect: Feeling keenly his lack of effectiveness in his environment, and galled by the resultant neglect, his primitive nature invites a paroxysm, which gains for him attentions, sympathy and other coveted advantages.

Inferior epileptics, in fact, usually have their attacks when subjected to some humiliating experience or neglect. It may be a fancied grievance, but to their hypersensitiveness, it is very real. The reality becomes unbearable, so they take refuge in an abnormal state which permits the freest expression to the untamed Caveman.

The physiological concomitance of many epileptic fits reflects an utterly primitive psychological state. The movements of the fingers, hands and arms may indicate a clawing, scratching design, or there may be recourse to savage thrusts, as of stabbing, or of a desperate strangling grapple with an imaginary foe.

That there has been an intuitive recognition of a dual personality in these cases, is evident from the fact that a person who raves or has a fit is said to be "*beside* himself." This descriptive term, like many other colloquialisms and slang words and phrases, displays significant accuracy and unconscious insight into a complex psychological situation.

### Hypnosis

Suggested sleep, or hypnosis, like the various pathological conditions described, is decidedly a split-off in the psychic stream. A study of this subject enables us to perceive the duality of the mind as by no other means. And it is particularly valuable in proving that the most casual experiences make a permanent photographic imprint on the unconscious mind even though this material is rarely available for conscious use.

Furthermore, in hypnotic states, we observe mental activities that are identical with some manifestations of insanity and with the more severe neuroses. Conscious reasoning ceases, but the unconscious mental processes are remarkably active. There is invariably a regression to an earlier age level, and unless the subject's talk is suggested by the hypnotist, it tends to revert to childhood memories. All idea of time disappears and the freedom from consciousness of time contributes much to the pleasure of the subject.

Every neurosis is essentially a form of unconscious auto-suggestion. The obsessive ideas of the neurotic are buttressed by what he holds to be very weighty evidence in the form of aggravating symptoms. And he develops an elaborate system of rationalization around them. The counterfeit nature of these symptoms, and their disappearance under the searchlight of understanding, have been noted.

The hypnotized subject who has performed some act or deed by direction of the hypnotist, will, if questioned, give very plausible reasons for so doing. Under the influence of the hypnosis, he cannot help doing it. He does it unconsciously, mechanically, and with unqualified certainty. But when the matter is brought into consciousness by questioning him, he rationalizes about it without knowing in the least why he does so.

An hypnotized subject may be told that at a certain time the next day he will call at a given address. Nothing further will be said about it. Upon coming out of the trance he will have forgotten all that transpired, but at the suggested time the following day he will call at the address specified. Having no real business there, he will unconsciously fabricate some "reason" for calling. He may say that he stopped to ask if the premises are for rent, or to inquire if a Mr.

So-and-so lives in the neighborhood, or anything else that seems plausible.

Luys mentions that he once heard a young married lady who had listened to one of his lectures, repeat the lecture several months afterwards in a hypnotic state, with the utmost accuracy, reproducing like a phonograph the very tone of his voice, using every gesture that he used, and adapting, too, in a remarkable way, her words to the subject. A year afterwards the lady had still the same capacity, and displayed it every time she was put into a trance. When awakened, however, she was utterly unable to repeat to him a single word of the lecture. She said she did not listen to it, that she did not understand a word of it, and could not say a single line.

This gives us an idea of the uncanny power of retentiveness of the unconscious mind, which the conscious mind is wholly unaware of, and is normally incapable of utilizing. It also illustrates what a marvellous factor suggestion is when it is applied so as to produce a psychic dissociation. When suggestion from another person will produce these amazing results, we are forced to realize that auto-suggestion, which is operative in every individual's life, must also have a powerful determining influence on our conduct. The great prevalence of neurotic subjects, with their endless array of counterfeited symptoms and ailments, is the commonplace expression of this phenomenon.

The positive influence of auto-suggestion in creative work must likewise be very great. The sensitiveness of persons of genius has been noted. The hallucinations some of them experienced were powerful auto-suggestions recorded on a hyper-sensitive imagination.

How many geniuses in perfecting their master-pieces could have been like Flaubert, who said that his characters seized upon him, and pursued him, or that, more correctly speaking, he lived through them? When he described the poisoning of Madame Bovary, he felt the taste of arsenic on his tongue, and showed symptoms of actual poisoning so far as to vomit.

## BIBLIOGRAPHY

JANET, PIERRE, *Major Symptoms of Hysteria*, New York, 1907.

BINET, ALFRED, *Somnambulism—Alterations of Personality*, New York, 1896.

SCRIPTURE, EDWARD W., *Stuttering and Lisping*, New York, 1912.

BLUEMEL, CHARLES S., *Stammering and Cognate Defects of Speech*, London, 1913.

FOREL, AUGUST, *Hypnotism or Suggestion and Psychotherapy*, New York, 1906.

QUACKENBOS, JOHN D., *Hypnotism in Mental and Moral Culture*, New York, 1903.

FOX, C. D., *The Psychopathology of Hysteria*, Boston.

HUDSON, THOMPSON J., *The Law of Psychic Phenomena*, Chicago, 1920.

# CHAPTER XVIII

## THE CAVEMAN CONCILIATED

On a sudden, in the midst of men and day,
And while I walk'd and talk'd as heretofore,
I seem'd to move among a world of ghosts,
And feel myself the shadow of a dream.
—TENNYSON, *The Princess.*

ALL the evidence of the foregoing chapters demonstrates two outstanding facts of the utmost importance to the individual's health and happiness. The first is the duality of personality—the elemental side being fundamentally primitive, and the intellectual side possessing widely varying rational and cultural possibilities. The second fact established is that the preponderance of human ills and ailments is due to a lack of working adjustment between these two energetic forces that constitute the mechanism of personality.

It therefore follows that the way to acquire a healthy organism (mental and physical) is to bring these two factors of the personality into harmonious relations. If there are severe, soul-torturing conflicts, they must, whenever possible, be traced down and eradicated by bringing them into the light of day. Another consideration of even more vital importance is to eliminate, as far as possible, the repressive agencies that tend to create the conflicts, especially in childhood.

### Relieving Psychic Disturbances

The experience of all the foremost exponents of psychotherapeutics has been that unconscious traumas may be healed, and their physical reflex-symptoms automatically eliminated, if the buried memories can be brought into consciousness.

This, when rightly understood, is neither mystical nor supernormal. It is perfectly natural and logical, as it represents the working of the law of hygiene and sanitation, which is operative in the psychic realm as well as in the material. Among the great achievements of science during the last century was the development of the principle of personal hygiene and social sanitation. It has been the supreme factor in reducing the ravages of disease and in substantially lowering the mortality rate.

The new psychology applies the same principle to the psychic sphere—and particularly to the deep, underlying region of the Unconscious, whose constant influence over us for good or ill we have stressed. No end of diseases, mental and physical, is caused by an accumulation of unhealthy psychic material below the threshold of consciousness. Emotional shocks in infancy or early childhood, that may have been due to excessive fear, worry or other cause which a rational, sympathetic explanation could have eased at the time, frequently leave their long-festering wounds. And these wounds, like those of the flesh, respond to hygienic, antiseptic treatment. They need psychic sunlight and intellectual oxygen.

An insight into the psychic processes is like the soothing sunshine that casts its health-giving rays upon the body and stimulates the vitality of every organ. A recourse to thought-provoking ideas, and cultivating the habit of inductive analysis, is the oxygen of the intellect, that keeps it clear, plastic and adaptable. An understanding of the mechanism of the emotions and the autonomic functions of the personality is the key to the dual goal of self-mastery and self-expression.

It was Dr. Breuer of Vienna, who about 1880, first struck upon the possibilities of removing deep-set psychoneurotic disturbances by relieving the mind of distressing, but unconscious, ideas. He called his system the "cathartic" method, which was well named, in that it indicated the purging of the mind of an incumbrance. This was a decided advance over the previous methods of the hypnotist who attempted to suggest the symptoms away.

Hypnotism, however, was in part responsible for Breuer's accidental discovery of the fact that the unconscious mind obtains relief by bringing to light its festering ideas. The patient whom he had hypnotized began to talk, while in the somnambulistic state, about the origin of the symptoms, and gradually a mass of forgotten circumstances connected with the seat of her trouble was reviewed.

The girl, who was suffering from severe hallucinatory hysteria, noticed that the symptoms disappeared as soon as their hidden casual connection was brought into consciousness. Breuer was shrewd enough to continue the treatment along the same lines—i.e., encouraging the patient to reveal the content of her subconscious mind, the "talking cure," she called it—until she was permanently free from all her hysterical symptoms.

It was, however, Breuer's colleague, Dr. Freud, who sensed the greater possibilities of the newly discovered psychic principle, which he took up with enthusiasm, and developed into a highly ramified science under the term, Psychoanalysis. His outstanding contribution has been in removing dream phenomena from the sphere of phantastic nonsense and placing them in the realm of abstract science.

All the experience of the psychoanalytic school has borne out the original contention that symptoms disappear when one has made their unconscious connections conscious. The most extraordinary and unexpected complications, however, are to·be met in the practical application of analytic treatment. It therefore necessarily follows that the effectiveness of the system is modified by the opportunities for reaching the repressed psychic material.

As the life experiences of the practitioner are different from those of the patient, it is evident that the former cannot remove the trouble by merely attempting to transfer his knowledge to the latter. The chief function of the analyst in the way of offering suggestions is to help the patient obtain a practical insight into his psychic operations. Beyond this, of course, he must be on the alert to seize upon any clues that may appear to have a bearing on the repressed idea-complexes, and to encourage the patient (as Breuer first did) to talk about them. In the desired state of abstraction, the subject will then tend to go deeper and deeper below the threshold of conscious mental activity, until the most remote regions of the psyche are plumbed and the obsessional ideas, by their exposure, rendered harmless.

### Childhood Problems

The prevalence of pernicious effects that are due to psychic traumas, mostly received in childhood, or that are later made possible by the irrational training of childhood, should emphasize the desirability of building early a foundation of mental health.

That there are serious economic barriers in the way of accomplishing this result among great masses of people is self-evident. That there are lamentable prejudices and other manifestations of ignorance that reinforce these barriers will not be gainsaid. The overcoming of these hindrances to racial health and human progress is a vast social and economic problem that space will not permit even touching upon here.

Nevertheless, there is a constantly increasing number of people who are honestly desirous of improving their own personality, and giving the fullest advantages of intellectual emancipation to their children. It is these people who will appreciate the newly recognized rights of childhood and the higher responsibilities of parenthood.

Child training of the past, and present, has been too largely a system of wholesale repressions, whereas *expression* is the law of life. If a healthy, wholesome outlet is not vouchsafed, then the "blocked" energy will simply break out in an individually or socially destructive form. It is this training which makes on the one hand the neurotic children and on the other the "bad" children.

The insubordinate child is a living protest against parental negativism. He is not encouraged along helpful lines that will develop his latent powers, and he receives only reprimands for his conduct, which grows increasingly mischievous. And in a sense he gains a form of substitute gratification, not only in his trouble-making, but in the chastisement itself. The primitive ego demands notice and consideration. It craves personal attention, which in a well-balanced childhood should be given by parents in the form of sympathetic counsel, helpful, stimulating suggestions and an abundance of actual coöperation. The boy (or girl) who abounds in vital energy, and is denied these balms of practical love, rather than soft sentimentality, finds that he does receive a flattering degree of notice when he commits mischievous acts. The thrill he derives from these exploits, which are invariably admired by his companions, and the attention he receives when caught, combine to emphasize his importance as an individual. He may be punished for some real or imaginary wrong-doing, but at least he has succeeded in asserting his individuality. Furthermore, he is something of a martyr in his own eyes. Most important of all, he has escaped the ignominious fate of the nonentity. He is a *personality.*

Severity towards and over indulgence of children are both inimical to the best development of their character. Constant criticisms tends to lessen a child's confidence in himself, and pampering weakens his initiative and resourcefulness. If carried to extremes, the result in either case may be ruinous. The mechanism of the personality that utilizes the energy is not sufficiently developed to dispose of the energetic force which the organism generates, so it blows off along some anarchistic, disorganized course. Thus comes the unadapted, and in time perhaps the unadaptable, personality. The legions who bear the hall-mark of futility and negativism are of this class.

Children should not be "forced" intellectually

beyond their years, with the idea of making prodigies out of them. Childhood should be a process of gradual, progressive growth, physical, emotional and mental, with full opportunities for an outlet of the playful side of the young, and not an attempt to cram the undeveloped mind with a mass of predigested information, greatly beyond its capacity for assimilation.

Knowledge should be imparted in such a way as to stimulate the child's intelligence, i.e., it should be presented attractively enough for him to desire to *grasp* it, instead of being *thrust* at him. Furthermore, his mind should not be balked by unnecessary inhibitions, nor choked by repressions or fears, but encouraged by training in the arts of expression, emphasizing those that are most in harmony with his particular mental bent.

Dr. C. W. Saleeby (*Parenthood and Race Culture*) states in regard to "education by cram and emetic": "Just so do we cram the child's mental stomach, its memory, with a selection of dead facts of history and the like (at least when they are not fictions) and then apply a violent emetic called an examination (which like most other emetics causes much depression) and estimate our success by the number of statements which the child vomits on the examination paper—if the reader will excuse me. Further, if we are what we usually are, we prefer that the statements should come back 'unchanged'—showing no signs of mental digestion.  We call this 'training the memory.' ''

Other educators who are far-sighted students of human nature have similarly expressed themselves, notably William Hawley Smith in his wise and inspiring book, *All the Children of All the People.*

## Power of Suggestion

The determining power of suggestion on each individual from earliest infancy is so far-reaching that its effects cannot be estimated.  Suggestion is at once glaringly obvious and indescribably subtle.  The form that results in unconscious imitation of behavior is perhaps much more influential in our lives than that consciously brought to bear upon us.  The latter often has its antidote in arousing the spirit of combativeness.  The manner in which it is presented may be offensive to one's ego, and therefore resisted.  There is no such opposition, however, offered to those suggestions which are unconsciously noted, and which become fixed habits through unthinking imitation and repetition.

Instinct itself, even in birds and animals where it is supposed to be quite paramount, is modified or thwarted when the environment lacks the element of suggestion conducive to normal development.

R. P. Halleck (*Education of the Central Nervous*

*System*), remarks, "If young birds are brought up where they cannot hear the song of their own species, they will never at a later time be able to sing the pure song of their kind."

This is only one of countless instances that might be cited of instincts that are frustrated, or native abilities that are atrophied, by lack of adequate environmental suggestion. The songbird that is raised away from its kind can never fully develop its wonderful singing qualities because there is missing the powerful element of suggestion—a satisfactory vocal model to imitate.

So it is that the child, too, from its first weeks of life begins to absorb impressions through its senses of perception. These are unconsciously noted, and with the infant's development, there is a growing evidence of its tendency to mimic— to respond to the suggestions that are constantly emanating from its environment.

As the child is the most imitative of creatures, it will mimic "bad" actions as well as "good"; improper speech as well as proper. And as there is more often a reaction of exceptional interest on the part of adults to questionable things that children say or do, the latter are quick to perceive that they have aroused unusual attention, and delight in holding this attention by following up the interesting lead they have struck through sheer imitation.

Neurotic children are literally bred in a neurotic environment as certainly as though neurotic nurseries were especially prepared for them. As the actions of a neurotic parent and others who may influence the child's life are apt to be either more interesting or more irritating than of those who are comparatively free from this affliction, the former are more likely to be imitated than the latter. The interesting and pleasingly eccentric traits are consciously seized upon and repeated, while the outstanding disagreeable or irritating actions are unconsciously repeated. In the course of time these subtle influences become ingrained into the character. So it is that the child who is a victim of such an environment suffers a handicap which may prove too great for him to overcome and he settles into an unadapted, neurotic adult.

The power of suggestion is utilized to an immeasurable degree in all schools of therapeutics and healing. This holds true from the most materialistic medical practitioner (whose pills and prescriptions in themselves are potent agents of suggestion), to those healing cults that treat human ailments exclusively by suggestion, although they may attribute their curative properties to some other cause.

The successful practitioner cultivates an atmosphere of cheerfulness so that his personality fairly radiates the suggestion of health. The influence of a personality of this type in a sick room is profound. At the same time, it is subtle, and therefore all the more effective. The influence operates on the unconscious mind to a far greater extent than on the conscious mind, because the latter is apt to feel too keenly the seriousness of the physical disability.

As the unconscious mind gets its impressions, not only in words, but more especially in pictures and symbolical representations, even a look of optimism and confidence will do much to effect a response of physical well-being. The physician's reassuring talk, and look of confidence regarding the patient's condition contribute a suggestion that impresses the patient with the belief in his recovery.

It is a very illuminating hypothesis regarding autosuggestion that has been advanced by Coué of the New Nancy School, and supported by much evidence of its effectiveness. In the past the *will* has undoubtedly been overemphasized as a direct influencing factor in our conduct, especially relating to health. Coué maintains that the will invariably yields to imagination, and that imagination is controlled and directed by autosuggestion.

### Coördinating the Psychic Powers

The alleged laziness of man has been held answerable for innumerable of his shortcomings. It is taken for granted in many quarters that man is ever anxious to shirk his duties, and therefore "human nature" has been roundly condemned. That he does often side-step responsibilities and duties is true, but might not some of the fault be with his training, his environment—even, in some instances, with the duties themselves?

If the facts cited in this book have proven any contention, it is that the human organism is a literal dynamo of energy. It is the natural function of this energy to express itself. The majority of the ills that afflict humanity is due to the failure of the complete organism to express itself adequately in a socially acceptable manner. When the energetic force is blocked or divided into conflicting currents, we have laziness, ineffectiveness, futility. We see the results, but do not realize the underlying cause.

Man, normally, is self-impelled to *action*. This characteristic of the race is more noticeable in children, who suffer less from blocked or diverted energy. The constant activity of a normal child is the marvel of all students of behavior. It is true that children do not like, and are injured by, the utilization of their energy in a routine manner. But the essential point is that they can, and do, express themselves tirelessly if permitted in a way that is adapted to their development at its various stages. That there is a sudden interruption of their psychic development in so many cases at the climacteric of adolescence is due to the fact that the natural, primitive outlet, which they had access to in childhood, is largely cut off, and society fails to offer a satisfactory substitute. For the want of a satisfactory substitute, they symbolically revert to the pleasing irresponsibility of childhood, shirk their work, and too often fritter away their time in injurious practices.

As William James has said, "Constructiveness is a genuine and irresistible instinct in man as in the bee or beaver." Actual laziness or inertia is an artificial habit inculcated by a pernicious environment. It is well known that prisoners have a horror of prison idleness. The lack of opportunity for normal expression of the personality, and particularly of the primitive side of the personality—the Caveman—is the chief cause of prison psychosis.

The monotony of stereotyped or routine occupations, which fail to give an adequate outlet to the desire for creative expression, is responsible for untold psychic discord, with all its hurtful potentialities. Work that is seemingly ineffective or vain becomes the height of drudgery, whereas the constructive endeavor of craftsmanship gives play to an emotional spring lying deep in the primitive nature of man. Veblen alluded to this when he said that man has " a taste for effective work, and a distaste for futile effort."

It is obvious from the material we have reviewed that the far greater part of the maladaptation of human beings to their environment is due to the lack of coördination between the primitive, unconscious desires and the conscious, socially trained ideals. And the latter are determined by each individual's particular environment, which is so often steeped in the negativism of repressions and inhibitions. Socially and industrially, ethically and educationally, the primitive personality—the Caveman—is balked and thwarted on all sides. Still, he is vital and in unnumbered instances may be rehabilitated and conciliated by considerate treatment—which is not more "rest," but greater opportunities for expression.

As has been previously stated, if one's occupation does not afford an adequate outlet for the ego urge or organic energy, then the personal interests should be broadened out until the gap is filled. In many cases, this is accomplished, to an extent at least, by activity in fraternal organizations or social movements. Again, the accumulating energy may be released in a highly beneficial way by taking up a hobby that offers free play to the creative instincts. Special, spare-time constructive work in the arts, music, literature or science is giving opportunities for expression to a constantly increasing number of people.

More people are capable of some socially useful and personally satisfying work along these lines than is commonly realized. Every one, except the hopelessly subnormal, has some degree of latent ability for creative endeavor. Jung remarked that he was always impressed when analyzing people by the enormous amount of artistic ability, repressed or undeveloped, that he found in his patients. That there is a coördination of conscious and unconscious processes in creative effort is plainly evidenced by the fact that there are required both the use of the rational faculties and the vital, autonomic energies of the emotional nature.

I can give no better illustration of the possibilities of successfully coördinating the psychic powers, with untold benefit to the physical organism, than to cite a case that has had my personal attention. The subject acknowledges receiving his only therapeutic help from my experience, and this fact, together with my intimate knowledge of his history, gives the fullest anthenticity to my observations.

The person in question, who is in his mid-thirties, had suffered from heart disturbances from childhood. At times the cardiac trouble was so pronounced that even the moderate physical effort required in his clerical duties quite exhausted him. He was considerably under-weight, and had been during all his adult years, was pale, suffered at times from extremely low blood pressure, and was subject to a form of anxiety neurosis. His anxiety and worries, which characteristically appeared to emanate from unconscious motives, were consciously concerned with his heart disability. There were times when even a short walk caused severe disturbances in the heart action.

The patient was studiously inclined, and

usually spent two or three hours each evening reading or writing. He had some small success in disposing of short stories and other literary work which he had taken up, but was advised by his relatives, on account of his chronic run-down condition and heart trouble, to give up the confining night work, and get more rest and sleep.

My observation of the case, from the subject's history, was that the trouble was not due to overwork, but to lack of psychic coördination, resulting in anxiety or worry, largely unconscious, and probably consciously associated with the distressing heart symptoms.

The first constructive suggestion was to acquaint him with the comparatively little danger from most heart disturbances as long as a few dietetic rules are observed, and physical excesses are avoided. In this case coffee was eliminated from the regular diet, although it might be drunk now and then, preferably not over a couple of times a week. As his occupation was sedentary, heavy, greasy foods were to be avoided as consistently as possible, and meat limited to once a day.

These minor regulations, which did not vary much from the patient's previous dietetic practices, were the only physical rules laid down. All other treatment was psychic. The subject was made acquainted with the details of the emotional mechanism and autonomic functions of the personality, and with the intricacies and interrelations of the conscious and unconscious mental processes. This enlightenment, which is covered by the subject-matter of the first half of this book and some of the later chapters, gave the patient a thorough insight into his organism as a whole, physical and psychic, in all its ramifications.

The understanding which he gained in the analysis of his unconscious conflicts relieved the long-standing physical symptoms. He has not been bothered by the former anxiety or worry, which he could hardly describe or define, but which was nevertheless very real.

As a result of the newly released energy, formerly consumed in internal conflicts, his health has been vastly improved and his efficiency increased many fold. Let us see what this coördination of the psychic energies has wrought.

In the year which has just elapsed as I write these lines, he has worked every day in a responsible position requiring a high degree of mental and physical energy. His duties are multitudinous and exacting. His hours, including commuting time, are long. He leaves home before eight in the morning and returns home about seven in the evening.

At night during this period of exactly one year, he has written three complete books, which have been highly praised by competent authorities who have read either the published work or the manuscript. During the same time he has read about fifty books, principally on scientific subjects, and written a number of special articles and book reviews for important periodicals. He is busy, and has been for the past twelve months, eighteen hours a day. His usual sleeping period is less than six hours.

What has been the effect physically of this strenuous work, made possible by harmonizing the psychic energies? He has gained fifteen pounds of healthy flesh, pulling him up from chronic underweight to normal weight for his height and age. His color has improved, all the functions of the body are operating better than in many years; and, most important of all, the *heart disturbances of many years' standing have disappeared.* Business friends, who are not acquainted with his private affairs, have complimented him on his healthy appearance, which has so greatly improved during the past year, and not infrequently they ask what "rest cure" he has taken.

A few concrete facts are often more illuminating than a whole library of theories, and so I have given a brief sketch containing the salient facts of an actual case. It is unnecessary to go into further details regarding this particular case because to an extent, each case is an individual one, with its own problems, difficulties and idiosyncrasies. However, the basis of almost all psychic and most physical irregularities is a lack of coordination of the mechanism of the personality —i.e., a conflict of greater or lesser degree between its primitive and intellectual components.

It is this highly complicated situation which the present volume, as a whole, attempts to analyze and clarify, and by so doing bring to the reader a real insight into the mechanism of his own personality. Just to that extent that the reader succeeds in seeing his inner self mirrored, he will to that degree be physically, mentally and spiritually benefited. He will find himself alienated from many of his ailments, and the efficiency of his energetic forces, creative powers and rational faculties correspondingly increased. All the functions of his personality will tend to become coördinated—the Caveman will be conciliated.

> Under the rules of correct reasoning, I have a right to assume that MAN HAS TWO MINDS.—THOMPSON J. HUDSON, *The Law of Psychic Phenomena.*

### BIBLIOGRAPHY

BRUCE, H. ADDINGTON, *Nerve Control and How to Gain It,* New York, 1918.

EVANS, ELIDA, *The Problem of the Nervous Child,* New York, 1920.

LAY, WILFRID, *The Child's Unconscious Mind,* New York, 1919.

SMITH, WILLIAM HAWLEY, *All the Children of All the People,* New York, 1919.

KEY, ELLEN, *The Century of the Child,* New York, 1916.

BAUDOUIN, CHARLES, *Suggestion and Autosuggestion,* New York, 1921.

BROOKS, C. HARRY, *The Practice of Autosuggestion* (by the Method of Emil Coué), New York, 1922.

THE END

# INDEX

.